Reiki for Beginners

Discover How to Improve your Energy, Reduce Stress, and Raise your Vibration with Reiki Healing. Start Now your Personal Awakening with Reiki Kundalini Meditation.

Table of Contents

Introduction

Chapter One: Introduction to Reiki

Chapter Two: Getting Started with Reiki

Chapter Three: Healing Yourself and Others with Reiki

Chapter Four: Chakras, Auras, and Energy Shields

Chapter Five: Reiki Lifestyle

Chapter Six: Reiki and Meditation

Chapter Seven: Testimonials and Stories

Conclusion

Introduction

These pages are packed full of information to help you get started on your Reiki journey. Whether you know nothing about Reiki, have already looked at a few beginner guides, or just know enough to have whet your appetite, you've come to the right place.

In the following chapters, you will learn about the history of Reiki and how it spread to the Western world. You will get an answer to the all-encompassing question: What is Reiki?

As you read, you will gain knowledge on how to use Reiki to heal yourself and others, as well as learning about energetic anatomy and energy systems in your body. You will discover how using Reiki can become a lifestyle, and as you progress through your studies, you will truly begin to live Reiki.

This journey will guide you through finding the best Reiki practitioner for yourself as well as using Reiki in meditations and meditations in your Reiki treatments. You will also read exclusive stories and testimonials from people just like you that have had amazing experiences with Reiki!

There are many books on the market that are about Reiki, so thank you again for selecting this book to be your guide. Although it is a beginner's guide, every effort was made to fill the pages with information and knowledge that are beneficial to your learning and Reiki practice. As always, enjoy the reading and good luck on your Reiki path.

Chapter One: Introduction to Reiki

What is Reiki? If you are just started out on your learning journey with Reiki and have no idea what Reiki really is, the simple answer is that Reiki is energy. Everything in the universe is infused with energy. Humans, as a whole, have been fascinated with this energy for centuries. Modern science measures it, tests it and has laws and theories about energy.

Reiki is the combination of two words 'Rei' and 'Ki.' The word 'Rei' translates into the word or concept of the universe. 'Ki' translates into energy, much like qui or chi. Reiki literally means Universal Energy. That is a very broad statement since everything in the universe is infused with energy, interacts with and responds to different energies.

A Reiki practitioner has the ability to become a conduit for Reiki energy and this is how Reiki treatments are performed.

So, what sets Reiki apart from other energy work practices? There are a few differences. One is that in order to become a Reiki practitioner and perform treatments, you must go through a Reiki Attunement ceremony in which a Reiki Master opens you up to receiving and giving Reiki.

Another major difference is that a Reiki practitioner becomes a one-way conduit for the Reiki energy. When you perform a treatment, you send energy through you, but you don't receive anything back. This means that as you perform a session on someone else, you get the benefit of Reiki and it doesn't tire you out because you aren't using your own energy.

Other differences with Reiki are that it can be performed with your hands on or hands off. It can also be sent over distances and time. Reiki is an intuitive therapy. The human body has an incredible capacity to heal itself. If the energy in the body is imbalanced, this creates unease in the body. Unease can then present itself as illness, injury, and disease. Reiki helps to amplify the body's natural ability to heal and rebalance the body's energy.

Oftentimes, if your body is in pain or you have an illness, the energetic imbalance that contributed to this manifestation of unease is completely unrelated to the actual problem. The source, if you will, of a headache, might be due to an energy block in an entirely different part of the body. Reiki being intuitive becomes a huge advantage.

As a practitioner, you don't necessarily need to know the source of the imbalance or unease. Reiki energy and the body work together to intuitively rebalance the systems and the body and heal the unease and present symptoms.

The uses for Reiki aren't just limited to healing yourself and others. Reiki can be included in many aspects of your life to enhance your lifestyle and maximize the balance and fulfillment you experience. This is yet another aspect that sets Reiki apart from other energy healing methods.

Reiki is a powerful energy work modality that works to intuitively create balance within yourself, others, and the environment and world you create for yourself.

History of Reiki

Reiki is a traditional Japanese style of energy work that was primarily passed down orally for centuries. Knowing the exact origins are difficult since the tradition was based on word of mouth for so long. However, Mikao Usui is credited as the founder of Reiki, as he rediscovered the art in the 1800s.

During a cholera epidemic in Tokyo, Usui fell ill, and while he was struggling to live and recover, he had a spiritual awakening. Once he was recovered, he was led to join a Zen monastery where he learned a healing method that had been used for centuries. This healing method includes laying static hand positions on the body. Usui did not dive directly into studying Reiki at this point, however, he wanted to increase his spiritual awareness of healing before continuing.

According to legend, he went on a spiritual quest which led him to a mountain top where he meditated and fasted for 21 days in order to better understand Reiki. He had a pile of pebbles with him while he meditated, and after each day, he threw one pebble away.

After the 21 days of meditation and study, Usui set a firm intention that he wanted to see things clearly. It is said that he received an energy flash the beamed straight through his forehead and supplied him with the Reiki Symbols that are used in Reiki treatments.

These were symbols that he had previously discovered in the Sutras he had been studying. It is believed that he reached enlightenment at this point in his studies.

As he traveled back down the mountain, he tripped and hurt his foot. The legend says he was bleeding and when he placed his hand over his foot, the cut stopped bleeding and the pain subsided. Then he stopped in a village and ate an entire meal without experiencing negative feelings or discomfort even though he had been fasting for 21 days.

When he returned to the Zen monastery, he used his new gift to heal the arthritis of his superior. Usui then decided to start using Reiki to try and help the poor and homeless communities in Kyoto. Unfortunately, he found that most of them would quickly return to their lifestyle of begging.

He was reminded that healing has to be holistic and includes the body, mind, and spirit. Usui returned to meditation and discovered the 5 principles of Reiki. Then he devoted the rest of his life to teaching and practicing Reiki.

Usui developed the teaching method of Reiki that included three degrees. The first degree, Shoden (first degree) was split into 4 levels: Loku – Tou, Go – Tou, Ton – Tou, and San – Tou. The second degree, Okuden (Inner Teaching) had 2 levels: Okuden – Zen – Ki (first part), and Okuden – Koe – Ki (second part). The third degree, or Master level, is called Shinpiden (Mystery Teaching). While there are 4 Reiki symbols, one being the Master Symbol, Usui only used three and did not teach the Master Symbol.

Another important contributor to the discovery and spread of Reiki was Chujiro Hayashi. A physician and retired Marine commander, Hayashi learned Reiki from Usui. Together, the two opened a Reiki clinic that combined Reiki with Hayashi's physician knowledge.

Hayashi kept detailed records at his clinic of what Reiki was used to treat and how different hand positions treated different conditions more effectively. With his notes and observations, he wrote the guide, *Reiki Ryoho Shinshin* which he included as a manual for students in his classes.

In his clinic, Hayashi expanded on how Reiki sessions could be given by developing the Group Session method. He would have a client lie on a table and multiple practitioners treat the client all at once. This created a much stronger energetic session. He also developed a new method for giving Reiki Attunements to his students.

Hayashi also changed the way that Reiki was taught. He would combine the Shoden and Okuden teachings and Attunements into one course, especially when he traveled. He traveled to Japan and was asked by his government to report on military information around Pearl Harbor.

Hayashi refused to provide such information and was dishonored by his government, being branded a traitor. To restore his family's honor, he performed seppuku or ritual suicide.

Howayo Takata is the woman who is most notably credited with bringing Reiki to America and the Western world in 1937. Takata was married to a bookkeeper at a plantation they both worked at in Hawaii.

After her husband died, it was her responsibility to support her family. However, after several years of hard labor and long work hours, she started to experience severe abdominal pain and problems with her lungs.

When her sister died, she was the one who had to travel to Japan and inform her parents, as they had resettled in Japan. While in Japan, she was admitted to a hospital and diagnosed with a tumor as well as gallstones. She was also diagnosed with asthma and appendicitis.

Rather than receiving surgery, Takata made her way to Hayashi's clinic for treatment. She had never heard of Reiki before, but the diagnosis she received at the clinic was very similar to what she got from the hospital, and this impressed Takata. She wanted to learn Reiki to keep healing herself and to bring it back to Hawaii with her.

For one year, Takata worked at the clinic and was taught by Hayashi. She was one of thirteen Reiki Masters trained by Hayashi. When she returned to Hawaii, she opened several clinics and started teaching Reiki. She would give sessions and treatments and taught students up to Level II Reiki.

Throughout the country and world, she was known as a healer.

In 1970, Takata began to offer the Master Level training for a cost of $10,000. Neither Usui nor Hayashi required a high fee for their teachings, however, Takata may have used the fee as a way to establish respect and legitimacy for Reiki practitioners. She believed that treatments and teachings should not be given for free.

During her courses, she did not provide written material or allow her students to take notes. Another deviation from Usui and Hayashi's teachings. The Reiki symbols were forbidden from being written down. She based her teaching methods off the ideology that Reiki was an oral tradition. She also insisted that a student must only work with one teacher during the studies.

Since these were deviations from the way Usui and Hayashi taught Reiki, it is not entirely clear why Takata had such restrictions for her students or charged such high fees.

By the time she passed away in 1980, Takata had taught and Attuned 22 Masters. These Masters began teaching their own students. Takata made them promise to teach the same way that she taught her students. However, after a time, Masters started relaxing their strict teaching methods and began allowing for notetaking and manuals. Students are now encouraged to seek out additional teachers to learn new methods and get different experiences.

Despite the exclusiveness of her teachings, Takata is still credited with how far and wide Reiki spread in the US and Western World.

Today, it is estimated that there are over 1 million Reiki Masters in the world and as many as 4 million practitioners. The more the scientific and medical fields find in regards to the human body and energy, the more interest there is in alternative methods such as Reiki. It has been used for centuries, even if not on a huge scale, so clearly it works!

As you progress through your own Reiki teachings, you will find many different avenues to study and receive Attunements. Some Masters will only teach in classes that might be a single weekend per Reiki Level. Other Masters might have developed online courses with all the information you need, and once you work through the course material, they will provide you with distance attunements.

Reiki has also expanded into several branches that have varying levels of learning and ways to practice. Usui Reiki is considered Traditional Reiki and that is going to be the basis of the information in this book.

Each Master has different course material and probably varies in the tasks and learning activities that you will be required to perform. The best you can do is find a Master that resonates with you and a learning style that you enjoy.

Five Principles of Reiki

When thinking of Reiki as a healing method, but also a lifestyle, we come back to Usui's five principles of Reiki. He discovered the five principles through meditation when he wanted to better understand how to incorporate body, mind, and spiritual healing with Reiki.

The five principles of Reiki are:

- For all of today, I will not worry.
- For all of today, I will not be angry.
- For all of today, I will work honestly.
- For all of today, I will be thankful for my blessings.
- For all of today, I will be kind to my neighbor and living things.

The human consciousness is fantastic at spinning stories in the mind that create anxiety, confusion, and suffering. The five Reiki principles are a great method for releasing those stories. Once released, each day can be faced with less stress and concern.

Releasing those stresses also create a more balanced and fulfilling life for yourself.

<u>For all of today, I will not worry</u>

Worry is an emotion that can be helpful in moderation, but in excess can be rather debilitating. If worry is abundant, the body and mind begin to experience problems with stress and anxiety. These high stress and anxiety levels begin to inhibit the healthy flow of energy in the body, eventually leading to unease and worse manifestations.

Worrying keeps your mind focused on the future, on what might be or could be. This takes your mind and consciousness out of the present. Small amounts of worry can be beneficial for making choices and leading to the future you want, but excessive worry builds confusion and inevitably creates stagnation.

The present, now, is the only time you are really effective. The only time you can really make a change and take action. Often, the struggles we experience help us become stronger or build our better future, so releasing worry and focusing on how you can change the present is going to inevitably build a better future.

To help release worry, make time every day to do something you enjoy or are passionate about.

<u>For all of today, I will not be angry</u>
Anger, like worry, can be helpful, but in excess becomes a hindrance. Usually, anger is the result of feeling helpless or like you have a lack of control or power. When a negative event occurs, our bodies often experience a strong emotional response. If that emotional response isn't released or isn't properly processed, it gets stored.

The next time we encounter a negative event that is similar to or reminds us of the original event, that stored emotion bursts out as anger.

Processing and releasing stored emotions a huge part of being a Reiki practitioner. Whether it is emotions within yourself or your clients. Unfortunately, society often frowns on expressing emotions, especially strong emotions like anger.

This makes it difficult to learn how to properly express and release emotions.

If you are feeling angry, breathe into the feeling. Take a step back and make yourself a witness to the situation rather than a participant. Taking yourself out of the situation gives you the chance to let the emotion pass rather than storing it.

<u>For all of today, I will work honestly</u>
Intuitively, our minds and bodies know when we are being honest. The subconscious tends to have a better understanding of our inner workings than our conscious mind. So if you are being dishonest with yourself, this can manifest as dissatisfaction, boredom, or resentment in one form or another.

Learning a life where you ignore your own dreams, goals, talents, and passions becomes a dishonest life. Making decisions based on fear rather than what you want will also lead to a dishonest life.

Every single person on the planet is important. Every single person has a role to play. How they live and what they do is going to resonate with the people around them and impact their environment and communities. Staying true and honest with yourself is how you are able to create the change that you are meant to create.

The dreams and passions you have are the universe's way of guiding you to the role you are supposed to play. Ignoring those isn't just detrimental to yourself, but it may create a rippling effect that affects others down the road.

Honor yourself, honor your dreams, and feed your passions. They will lead you to where you should be.

<u>For all of today, I will be thankful for my blessings</u>
It is so easy to allow the ego to see all events as either good or bad, black and white. When looking at events with the soul and not the ego, the consistency changes. Every experience is a learning opportunity or a message. Choosing what you want to take away from the experience is how it is going to define you for better or worse.

There is a heavy emphasis on searching outside of ourselves for happiness and fulfillment. Once you accept that happiness and joy must come from within, the entire world changes! If you can focus on how to create your own happiness and fulfillment within yourself, experiences don't look so black and white anymore. Reaching for what you don't have no longer seems to be the answer to fulfillment.

Changing yourself changes your environment. Having gratitude changes the vibration of your body, mind, insights, and wisdom. You have countless things in your life to be grateful for. Coloring life in a light that has gratitude can change how your eyes see the world, how your mind processes events, and how your emotions respond to events.

<u>For all of today, I will be kind to my neighbor and living things</u>
Since the human body is infused with energy, and science tells us that energy has waves and frequencies, the human body gives off an energetic

frequency or vibration. When you put out a specific energy frequency, you are likely to draw in people and events that have a similar energy vibration.

The intention is powerful. There have been many studies on the water that show water molecules exposed to negative energies, thoughts, and words are drastically different than water molecules that have been exposed to positive thoughts, words, and energies. This difference can be measured at a molecular level! The human body is comprised of a large amount of water, therefore, the water molecules in the human body are subject to the same impact.

The people around us become mirrors for ourselves. If you choose to be kind, helpful, and reflective, you will begin to see those changes in the people around you as well. Choose a life of peace and satisfaction; that is your greatest responsibility to yourself.

The five Reiki principles can be incorporated into your life in any way that you see fit. Whether you include them in meditation, speak them aloud, or write them down, they have the power to keep changing your life. Usui used them as the basis for spiritual and mental healing which lends a hand to the physical body healing.

If you are not already familiar with meditations or affirmations, start using the five Reiki principles as affirmations. Start practicing mediations that include Reiki principles. If you are already familiar with meditations and affirmations, find a way to incorporate the 5 principles into what you already use.

Taking the next step as a Reiki practitioner can be a commitment, but it doesn't have to be. Moving through the teachings step by step, you can decide how far you want to go and how much you want to invest in the learning.

Step by Step Reiki Learning Process

<u>Reiki Level I (Shoden)</u>

Reiki Level I is the first degree of Usui Reiki. While each Master and teacher will vary their training, generally, the first degree follows a typical pattern of teaching.

You'll learn:

- What Reiki is
- History of Reiki
- Self-treatment hand positions
- Hand positions for treating others
- Reiki Principles and Pillars
- Energetic Anatomy
- Reiki Applications

After progressing through the course work, you will likely receive tasks to complete such as reading assignments and assessments. Once the course work is completed, you'll receive your Reiki Level I Attunement.

The Attunement process is a ceremony that the Master performs to open the student up to give and receive Reiki. It connects them to the energies of

Reiki and allows them to begin practicing Reiki on themselves and others.

Next, you will want to:

- Perform 21 Reiki sessions on yourself over 21 consecutive days
- Perform 21 consecutive Reiki sessions on someone else over 21 consecutive days (the same person or different people is acceptable)

This 21-day treatment period may not be required by your Master, however, it is symbolic of Usui's 21 days of meditation while he was learning about Reiki and progressing on to learning the Reiki Symbols which are revealed in Level II Reiki.

You'll study applications of using Reiki in everyday life and learn about the energetic bodies like chakras and auras as well as how Reiki works with the body.

Reiki Level II (Okuden)

Second degree Reiki is when you will learn about the Reiki symbols that can be used to enhance treatment and amplify Reiki energy. If you do plan on providing Reiki as a service for others, it is recommended that you at least complete the Level II training. While it isn't required, Level II brings you into a deeper connection with Reiki and energy healing.

You'll learn:

- Three Reiki power symbols
- Performing distance Reiki sessions
- Performing Reiki sessions through time
- Reiki meditations
- Enhanced techniques for Reiki sessions
- Advanced Reiki techniques (such as Reiki for animals or Crystal Reiki)

Different courses may include different variations of the advanced Reiki techniques, or offer them as separate courses altogether. Three of the Reiki power symbols will open up your ability to use Reiki across time and space, thus opening the door for providing distance Reiki treatments.

Since you will be deepening your connection to Reiki during this level, learning about different meditations for Reiki and how to include those meditations and techniques into your sessions is going to be included at this level.

Once you complete the reading assignments, assessments, and tasks from Level II Reiki, your Master will perform your Level II Attunement.

After receiving your Attunement:

- Perform 5 Reiki sessions on yourself with symbols over 5 consecutive days
- Perform 5 Reiki sessions on someone else with Reiki symbols over 5 consecutive days (the same person or different people is fine)
- Perform 5 distance Reiki session over 5 consecutive days

Again, these steps may not be required for your specific class, but it helps you learn how to incorporate Reiki symbols into your session and get a better handle on using your different Reiki tools.

Reiki Master Level (Shipiden)

The Reiki Master Level is going to vary greatly depending on who you learn from. This may be the level that includes some advanced Reiki techniques as well.

Not everyone decides to progress to the Master Level. That is fine, you will want to progress as far as you feel called to. The Master Level isn't required if you are just using Reiki as a service, but if you want to start teaching Reiki, this is the level you will want to reach.

You'll learn:

- The Master Reiki Symbol
- Alternative or non-traditional Reiki Symbols
- Reiki Attunement Ceremonies
- How to perform and Attunement ceremony

- Variations on the Attunement Ceremony
- Distance Attunement Ceremonies
- Advanced Reiki Techniques and Consciousness levels

After completing the course work and assignments, you will receive your Master Level Attunement and hopefully have the opportunity to practice and Attunement Ceremony with your Master.

As always, the course material may vary depending on the Master that you are learning form. Some may not teach distance Attunements if they only use in-person Attunements themselves.

Regardless, the Master Level is going to give you deeper access to Reiki, energy, and your own consciousness. You will also greatly expand on how you perform sessions. Some Masters will perform all the Attunements at once, and then you can progress through the coursework at your own pace. Other Masters might offer a combined Level I and II course and attunements.

There is always more information to expand on your Reiki knowledge. You may decide to seek out multiple Masters and teachers to help you deepen your knowledge. You may start with Level I and not feel the need to progress onto the next level for many years. Work at your pace and respect your intuition as it guides you.

Chapter Two: Getting Started with Reiki

When you are first getting started with Reiki, it is best to find a Master/Teacher that you are going to gain the most from working with. Does this mean the Master with the most experience? Does it mean the Master with the most students? Does it mean the Master who has been teaching longest?

You may want to think about your own learning style. Do you want to take an in-person class with other students, or do you want to take an online course that you can work through at your own pace? Maybe you are looking more for one-on-one mentorship with a Master?

Some questions to ask yourself when searching for a Reiki teacher:

- Do you want in-person classes?
- Do you want online classes?
- Do you want a teacher that is easy to contact?

- Do you prefer working at your own pace?
- Are you a visual or hands-on learner?
- How much time do you want to devote to learning?
- How much time do you have to devote to work, family, school, etc?
- Do you want a one-on-one learning experience?
- Are you willing to travel for your studies?

Most cities now do have local Reiki teachers that offer different kinds of classes. Beyond that, there are plenty of online courses available now for Reiki as well. Doing a quick online search can help you find the local courses available in your area, or even lead you to some online sources.

Since Reiki is energy work, you are going to want to find a teacher or Master that you feel you resonate with. Think of it like when you are looking for a doctor. If you meet a new doctor that asks you uncomfortable questions or talks too much about their personal lives, you may end up looking for a different doctor as well.

Your Reiki Master is going to be working with you on a personal level. This is physical, emotional, spiritual, and energetic. You are going to want a practitioner that you feel you can trust and that you want to learn from.

Learning Reiki should be a pleasurable experience. It should be interesting, engaging, and keep you wanting to learn more. That being said, sometimes, very well-known Reiki practitioners might be hosting a weekend course in a specific area. If learning from the well-known Masters is what you want, you may have to set time aside to travel to where they are hosting their classes.

Listen to your intuition. If you are working in-person with a practitioner, see if you can talk to them beforehand and gauge during the conversation if you think that they will be a good fit for you to work with.

Even Reiki Masters and Teachers have different energy frequencies, so you should take the time to find a Master that is going to offer you the best learning experience, which only you can determine for yourself.

If you plan on providing Reiki as a service to others and perhaps even starting your own Reiki practice, then you'll want to consider some of the tools you may want to acquire or invest in.

Having a massage table to perform Reiki sessions on is a great idea! Not only are they designed for your client to be comfortable lying supine and prone, but they make for more ergonomic positioning for you as you work down the body with hand positions.

Designating a space for practicing Reiki is also a good idea. Whether it is a rented space or in your home, if you are going to be seeing clients, having a Reiki space will help with the energy, healing, and overall professionalism. Decorating a space to inspire relaxation and peace can improve the atmosphere of a Reiki session.

That doesn't mean you can't provide mobile Reiki services the same way as some massage therapists provide mobile massage.

Overall, the most important tools you will need for Reiki are your hands and the Reiki symbols. Once you've received your attunements, your hands and the symbols are going to be your primary resource in performing sessions and treatments. Take care of your hands.

The second most important tool for you when working with Reiki is your intuition. Intuition is going to help guide your healing hands. If you feel like you aren't connected with your intuition, start developing it because you will need it as a healer.

Some additional tools that practitioners will include in sessions are:

- Singing Bowls
- Aromatherapy
- Hot Stones
- Toning

- Crystals

Singing Bowls and toning do fall into the same category of sound therapy. You don't need formal training to use singing bowls or vocal toning, however, it is recommended if you want to make it a regular part of your sessions.

Aromatherapy is a great way to enhance Reiki sessions either with the use of essential oils on the skin or through diffusing essential oils into the air. Again, if you would like to use essential oils on your client's skin, getting formal training is recommended.

Hot stones are a lovely addition to a Reiki session as they really enhance the relaxation process as well as reduce tension in the muscles. If you are going to use hot stones, definitely look into formal training options as if used incorrectly they can cause painful burns and damage to your clients. When used correctly, they are a wonderful enhancement to Reiki sessions.

Crystals are another favored tool in Reiki. Crystal Reiki is even offered as its own course with its own Attunement. Crystals are a naturally-occurring, highly stable, mathematically constructed energetic catalyst. The crystalline matrix of firmly set molecules has an impressive capacity to store, absorb, refract, transmute, and reflect light. This is what gives crystals their unique colors and properties.

If you are unfamiliar with crystals in energy work, it is a whole other world that you are encouraged to explore.

Just like Reiki, crystals have been used for thousands of years in healing. As far back as ancient Egyptian civilizations, crystals were prescribed as medicine. Patients were told to carry certain crystals with them or wear them in an effort to heal a disease or pain.

In modern science, what that means is that crystals all resonate at a different energetic frequency. By holding that energetic frequency on our bodies, our own frequency will begin to change to match the crystal.

Crystals have been used in ancient Chinese medicine being ground up and actually added to tonics. Their use around the world was popular up until medieval times when science and medicine started to turn away from 'archaic' traditions and looking more at 'fact-based' treatments. Crystals began to resurface in popularity in the seventies and interest and popularity keep growing.

Of course, modern science can and does now explain the energy of crystals and how they interact with the human body. Different instruments can actually measure the energetic output and resonance of crystals.

Becoming more accepted as an alternative therapy, just like Reiki, crystal availability and knowledge is becoming more available. Some crystals do have toxic components, so if you would like to use crystals, make sure that you understand their properties and which ones shouldn't be placed directly on someone's skin.

Crystals, on their own, are fantastic energy healing tools that naturally amplify Reiki energy. Reiki, on its own, is a great energy healing tool that can provide more structure to crystal healing. They are mutually beneficial when used in combination.

Crystal Reiki implements the use of crystal grids, which are geometric shapes that are built out of crystals. These grids can be placed directly on a client or under the table or chair they are lying or sitting on. You can learn crystal properties fairly easily, but your intuition is also going to be a major factor when you start making crystal grids.

One huge advantage of using crystals with Reiki is that the crystals can be used to target specific ailments with Reiki energy. Reiki is an intuitive modality, and as previously touched on, it tends to go where it needs to go and balances what it needs to balance, regardless of if the practitioner is aware of what needs to be fixed or not.

When combining crystals with Reiki, you gain the advantage of being able to work on specific body parts and ailments.

Crystals don't have to be used in grids though. A single crystal can be added to a Reiki session or charged with Reiki energy to help enhance a session. There are thousands of crystal types that naturally occur in the world. Depending on their color, shape, geometric matrix, and inherent properties, they can resonate powerfully with specific qualities.

These qualities can then be enhanced and drawn out with the Reiki energy.

Many Reiki practitioners like to combine crystals with their energy work. There is plenty of information on using crystals in healing, but if you want to pursue it more seriously, look for a Master or Teacher that has Crystal Reiki experience.

Three Pillars of Reiki

The three pillars of Reiki are essentially a tool that you can use in Reiki and your Reiki sessions. It is said that Usui used these three pillars in his own sessions. The three Reiki pillars are methods of meditating with Reiki energies that can be used to deepen your connections to Reiki energies and healing.

The three pillars of Reiki are:

- Gassho (Meaning: Two Hands Coming Together)
- Reiji-Ho (Meaning: Reiki Power Methods)
- Chiryo (Meaning: Treatment)

Gassho

Pronounced Gash-Show is a Reiki meditation taught to help hold the intention of gratitude, focus, respect, balance, and a connection to consciousness.

To perform a Gassho meditation, you start by putting your hands together in a prayer position in front of your chest, palms flat together, and fingers straight. Gassho should be performed in a seated position.

Once you have the position, you want to bring your awareness to the tips of your middle fingers, holding your awareness there. Any time that your mind starts to wander, press the tips of your middle fingers together and refocus your awareness.

When you first start Gassho meditations, you may find it hard to stay focused. Start practicing in 3-minute intervals, slowly increasing the amount of time in which you meditate.

There are two types of Gassho meditations. There is an informal meditation and a formal meditation.

Formal Gassho meditations are traditionally used in ceremonies. This can include religious ceremonies, although Reiki has no religious affiliation. With Formal Gassho, you will put your palms together in prayer position. From there, you will raise your elbows, holding your arms at about

30 degrees to the floor. You'll want your fingertips at the height of your eyebrows and your hands about four inches away from your nose. You'll keep your eyes focused on your fingertips.

The informal position for Gassho is slightly different and called Mu-shin, meaning 'no mind.' In Mu-shin, your fingertips will be lightly touching, but your palms will be slightly separated. Hold your forearms at a 45-degree angle to the floor. You'll still want your hands about four inches from your face, only in this position, your fingertips will be just below your nose. Your eyes will stay focused on your middle fingers. Mu-shin is commonly used for greeting others.

If this meditation is beneficial to you, it is recommended that you perform it every day. In the morning and at night if possible. Additionally, when you meditate, taking notes on your own experiences can be helpful, especially when you are first starting out.

To perform a Gassho Meditation:

- In a seated position, place your hands in the Mu-shin Gassho position. Sit in a chair or on the floor.
- Focus your eyes on where your middle fingers meet.
- Let all your thoughts melt away. If thoughts start to arise in your mind, let them go, watch them pass, and keep your focus on your middle fingers.
- Speak the five Reiki principles aloud.
- If your arms start to get tired, slowly lower your hands to your lap.
- Any sensations you begin to feel, allow them to pass as well.
- When you have finished, set an intention of gratitude.
- If you need to, ground yourself by placing your palms on the floor or holding a grounding crystal.

<u>Reiji – Ho</u>

Pronounced Ray-Gee-Ho, the word Reiji means 'the indication of Reiki power' and the word Ho means 'technique.' Reiji-Ho is three short rituals that can be performed before or alongside Reiki sessions to enhance the session and bring you deeper into the healing.

Step One:

- Hold your hands out in front of your chest in the Gassho position and close your eyes.
- Using the Reiki symbols, as that Reiki energy flow through you.
- Repeat this request or intention three times.
- Then activate the CKR and SHK Reiki symbols to hold your intention.

Step Two:

- Ask for the client or recipient to receive balance during their session.
- Keeping your hands in the Gassho position, raise them to your Third Eyes chakra.
- Ask to have your hands drawn to or guided to where the Reiki energy is needed.

Step Three:

- Allow the Reiji-Ho technique to guide your hands over your client.
- Detach your mind from any desires or expectations that you might have for the outcome of the treatment session.
- Be open to receiving any visions or messages that will help guide you through the session.
- Once Reiji-Ho is complete, your hands will stop moving or be still.
- Perform the Gassho one more time.
- Perform a regular Reiki session with a little extra focus on the areas designated by Reiji-Ho.
- You can choose to discuss what you discover with your clients or not.

<u>Chiryo</u>

Pronounced Chi-Rye-Oh, Chiryo in English means 'treatment.' To perform Chiryo, you, as the practitioner, will place your dominant hand above your client or recipient's crown chakra. When you receive a signal to move, start moving your nondominant hand over their body as your intuition guides you.

Your intuition will guide your hand placement, how long each position is held, and the other aspects of the session. Once you are called to end the session, do so.

You can use Chiryo alongside a traditional Reiki session or as its own treatment session.

The three pillars of Reiki can be used to deepen your own connection with Reiki as well as strengthen your intuition and make a treatment session stronger. Take the time to practice each method and see if they work for you or what resonates with you.

Reiki as an energy therapy does work with the physical body. The physical body being skeleton, muscles, organs, circularity system, lymphatic system, reproductive system, etc. Reiki also works closely with the Chakra and Aura systems of the body. Two energetic systems of the body.

Chakras and Auras will be discussed in later detail in another chapter, however, both systems create energy fields in and around the body. This energy can become imbalanced just like the rest of the body and can lead to unease.

There is a common school of thought among energy workers, including Reiki practitioners, that if the body maintains perfect energetic health, then the body maintains perfect physical health.

For example, an energy blockage in a certain portion of the body could create an energy deficient muscle. When the muscle weakens because it isn't receiving the proper energy flow, then that muscle is going to be more easily damaged, torn, strain, or injured.

Everything within the body is connected. This includes the physical parts of the body, mental processes in the body, and the energetic fields of the body. Reiki works on all three levels and this is one of the many reasons it is so powerful at balancing and aligning the body to perfect health.

So what about Reiki and anatomy?

Since the body is intuitive on its own and since Reiki is intuitive on its own, as the practitioner, you are merely the catalyst that shifts Reiki energy from the universe into someone else. By providing that energy to them, their body is able to balance and heal itself.

Having a basic knowledge of anatomy and physiology will help you better understand common ailments and issues. You may not be able to direct the Reiki energy specifically, but when working with clients, having that knowledge will allow you to speak to them more professionally. You can also offer them additional suggestions with their Reiki treatments.

Systems that can be highly benefited by Reiki include:

- Endocrine System
- Lymphatic System

- Reproductive System
- Nervous System

This isn't to say that Reiki can't benefit all the systems. However, the Endocrine system is all the glands and hormones in the body. Hormones regulate just about everything in the body. From growth, metabolism, sex drive, and development of organs.

Thyroid imbalances are common and cause all kinds of immune system and health issues.

Reiki as a treatment can balance the production and distribution of hormones as well as balance the glands themselves. Overproduction and underproduction of hormones can result in health issues throughout the body.

If something is being overproduced or under-produced, it is imbalanced. Therefore, Reiki can be the treatment to recreate balance and health in the endocrine system.

The lymphatic system is part of the circulatory system and the immune system. Lymphatic veins move a fluid called lymph through the body. Lymph is vital for fighting any viral and bacterial infections. Lymph nodes are a station in the body where those viral and bacterial infections are addressed.

There are large clusters of lymph nodes in the neck, chest, armpits, elbows, abdomen, groin, knees, and ankles.

The Lymphatic system includes the thoracic duct in the chest and the spleen. Unlike the circulatory system, there is no pumping organ that pushed lymph through the veins. Movement of the body is what stimulates lymph flow.

When lymph stops flowing and gets blocked, it can create a swelling called lymphedema. Patients being treated for various stages of cancer also have to take a close look at their lymphatic system.

As a balancing treatment, Reiki can greatly improve lymphatic flow and health. It is not a body system that is well-known or talked about, but it is vital and Reiki works very well with the lymphatic system.

When it comes to the reproductive systems, this seems to be one of the most sensitive systems in the body, especially for women. In this day and age, so many chemicals and GMOs and artificial hormones are thrown at women that infertility levels are rising as well as birth defects and mental health disorders that can be linked with reproductive health.

While Reiki isn't a cure-all, if there is a problem with the reproductive system, it often has to do with an imbalance of some kind. This can be an overabundance of a hormone or an under abundance of a hormone. More drastically, it could be the presence of high levels of a toxic element, such as mercury.

While they may not be debilitating, it may not become apparent that there is an imbalance until conception is attempted.

Many women who have struggled with infertility and have gone through fertility treatments have also decided to use Reiki alongside their treatments and have found success with it!

Reiki helps with infertility on multiple fronts. First of all, it will begin to address imbalances in the body that can help conception be achieved.

Women who are struggling with infertility or who might be currently undergoing fertility treatments may be experiencing a lot of physical and emotional pain. Reiki can help relieve physical pain as well as release emotional pain.

When the body feels healthy and the mind is in a healthy state, then that can create an environment of wellness which will also contribute to the effectiveness of fertility treatments.

Again, we can see how Reiki affects different levels of anatomy in physical, mental, and energetic to provide balance and wellness.

The nervous system controls everything in the body. Every muscle, organ, vein, gland, everything has attachments to the nervous system. The nervous system connects the brain to the rest of the body and keeps the body functioning. More than that, the nervous system runs off of electrical impulses.

What is electricity if not energy? Slight impairment of energetic flow in the nervous system can start a chain reaction through the whole body that might result in an entirely different issue. Correcting the nervous system imbalance can realign the rest of the issues.

If the human body runs off the nervous system, and the nervous system is electrical energy, then it makes sense that Reiki energy can be a powerful asset to nervous system health.

Nerves in the body can be quite sensitive and be thrown out of balance easily. If you've ever experienced a tingle in your arm because you haven't moved it in a while, this is your nerves telling you that you aren't getting enough blood to that area of the body. If you've ever stubbed your toe and felt pain when walking, this is your nervous system telling you that you injured your toe and not to put pressure on it.

Headaches are the brain's response to an over firing, under firing, or misfiring of electrical, neurological impulses. If you've ever had a headache or migraine where the part of your head that hurts is physically swollen, that is usually because there is a misfiring of the nerves and it is creating a painful response in the brain. Misfiring is just another term for imbalanced.

So you can see that an energy work method like Reiki can resonate strongly with the nervous system.

When you are first starting out with your Reiki journey, remember to find a practitioner and teacher that you really resonate with, one who will provide you with the best learning experience for yourself. You want this teaching process to benefit you at its highest.

While additional tools aren't required for Reiki, there are some that might enhance your sessions or help you establish a practice. If you do plan on performing Reiki on others, having a massage table is highly recommended.

The three Pillars of Reiki are three energetic tools that you can use when treating others or when treating yourself with Reiki. You can also incorporate the five principles of Reiki into the three pillars to really start living Reiki.

The body and all the body systems, whether they are physical or energetic, are infused with energy. This energy is what Reiki balances to ensure a healthy, balanced body and life. The more you learn in your studies and the more you begin embracing your Reiki lifestyle, you will start to see the changes in yourself and around you. Some of the changes are very subtle and you might not notice them for a while. But even the subtle changes are important.

When you are just getting started and figuring out how Reiki fits in your life and what you want to do with it, try keeping a journal. Write down your experiences with your Master, or what you feel when you receive sessions. Take notes on self-treatment and our meditations. Eventually, you will be able to look back on what you took notes on and see how far you've come.

Note-taking can also help you develop your intuition. Writing down visions, feelings, sensations, and anything else you experience during sessions, Attunements, and meditations is a great way to help you start to understand how that information relates back to you. The more you practice, the less you will find the need to write things down in order to translate them for yourself.

Energy resonates with energy. Energy reacts to energy. Science says that energy cannot be created or destroyed, only transformed. This is exactly what Reiki does. Reiki doesn't remove blocks or create more energy in the body. It transforms the energy

that already exists in the body to achieve a naturally
healthy and balanced state.

Chapter Three: Healing Yourself and Others with Reiki

Self-Treatments

When you first start learning Reiki, you are going to be wanting to perform Reiki treatments on yourself. As you progress through your studies, make self-Reiki treatments part of your daily routine.

A self-Reiki treatment doesn't have to be long, however, getting in the habit of giving yourself a 20 to 40-minute Reiki treatment every day is going to yield the best results. As a practitioner, the first goal you should have is to improve yourself. Improving yourself is going to allow you to improve your environment, your world, and also allow you to better heal others.

A short self-Reiki treatment could be as simple as placing your hands on your head and performing Reiki for five minutes. These shorter Reiki treatments are best used throughout the day if you have a headache or need to help yourself refocus. Performing a full self-treatment at a designated time is best.

When you perform a self-treatment, you'll be holding static hand positions on yourself for 3 to 5 minutes each. You can use a designated set of hand positions, develop your own hand positions, or just intuitively place your hands where you are called to place them.

To prepare for a self-Reiki treatment, make sure you can designate 20 to 40 minutes of time alone and undisturbed. If you have a meditation space or intention space, that can be a great place to perform your self-treatments.

You can either be sitting or lying down for a self-treatment. Although a common result of Reiki is to feel so relaxed you fall asleep, so if you have obligations set for after your self-treatment, you may want to be sitting.

You'll want to create a relaxing and peaceful atmosphere. Whether that is through dimming the lights, playing relaxing music, or lighting some candles and incense, set the mood for yourself.

Generally, when you perform a Reiki session, you'll want to start from the head and work your way down.

Not only do self-treatments give you the chance to heal yourself, but you also get to practice Reiki daily. Your intuition will also start to develop. That way, if you decide to offer Reiki services or perform them on other people, you might better be able to answer their questions.

For example, if someone comes to you who have never had Reiki before and they want to know what it will feel like, having performed Reiki on yourself, you can explain to them some of the sensations they might feel.

Albeit, everyone experiences Reiki differently, but if you give them something to consider, that is better than leaving it vague and too open.

Once your mood is set and you get yourself comfortable, you'll start your hand positions. The picture below gives a rough outline of hand positions you can use on yourself in Reiki treatments.

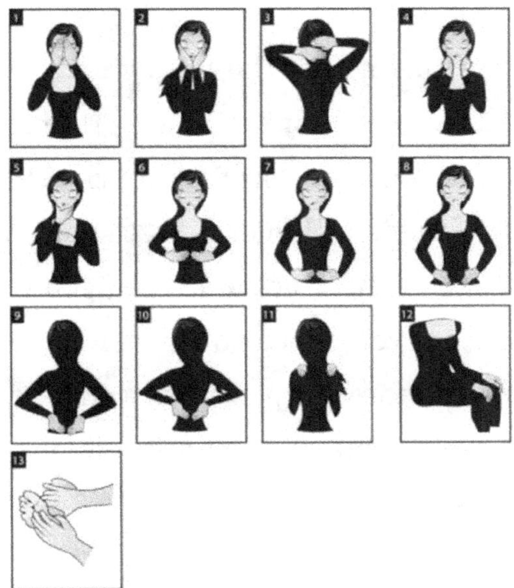

If you are new to Reiki, it isn't a bad idea to start with these hand positions. Once you get more comfortable with your intuition and Reiki energy, you'll be able to change positions, add positions, or just follow your own intuition as you feel called.

During a self-treatment, some practitioners find that they like to start and/or end with a Gassho meditation. You may also like to start or end by touching each of the seven main chakras on your body (more information will be given about chakras in a later chapter).

During a self-treatment, breathe deeply and clear your mind. Practice mindfulness, being present in that moment. Also, practice conscious touch, which is being fully in the moment that you are performing Reiki. Conscious touch is good to practice, especially if you plan on offering Reiki as a service. One of the poorest experiences a client can have is if they get on your table and feel like your mind isn't focused on the session.

What this means is when you are performing a Reiki session, whether it is on yourself or someone else, don't be thinking about what you're going to make your dinner, if the dog got let out, or when you have to pick your kids up from school. Keep your mind centered on the session and the person you are working on, even if it is yourself.

When you perform a self-treatment it is not uncommon for heavy emotions to surface. If you find yourself feeling a strong or heavy emotion, let yourself feel it. Let yourself release that emotion during the session. Hold the hand position you have for that emotion and don't move to the next hand position until you have fully released the emotion.

Especially when you are first starting out, try writing some of your experiences down. Each Reiki session is unique and everyone feels Reiki differently. Your skin might tingle or feel warm, your breathing pattern might change. You might feel sensations or emotions that you aren't used to. You can even get visions and ideas during a session.

Universal energy is a vast source of wisdom and knowledge. That information can be downloaded, just like on a computer. Instead of going onto a hard drive, universal downloads end up in our minds and bodies. It can take a little practice deciphering the meanings behind some of the things you experience.

Therefore, writing it down and allowing yourself the time and space to analyze it will add a deeper connection to yourself and your Reiki treatments. Symbols you receive are going to be personal to you. You could see a butterfly and know exactly what it means to you, yet a butterfly could have an entirely different meaning for someone else.

It is worth noting that if you do fall asleep during a self-treatment; when you wake up, pick up the treatment where you left off to finish it. Or, if you don't have the time, the next self-treatment you perform, start where you last remember leaving off before falling asleep and then complete a full session.

Self-treatments can be personal and private, so don't feel like you need to share what you experience. If you do have questions, your Master should be able to help guide you with those questions. The sooner you can get into the habit of daily Reiki treatments on yourself, the better, especially during your studies and your early practice days.

Treatments on Others

Of course, many Reiki students are taking Reiki courses because they want to learn how to perform sessions on other people.

A Reiki session being performed on someone else is going to be similar to self-treatments but do tend to be more involved. Your clients can either sit in a chair or lie down on a table. Generally, a full session performed on someone else is going to take 45 minutes to an hour. Sometimes, they can be 90 minutes or 120 minutes. This is partially going to be based on what you want to offer clients. Standard time is 45 minutes to 1 hour.

When designating a location for Reiki sessions, try to ensure a peaceful and tranquil environment. This can often mean low lighting, limited natural light, and an appropriate temperature level. Not too hot and not too warm. You can also provide blankets and sheets for table sessions.

A client does not need to get undressed for a Reiki session, so you don't have to supply sheets, but having a blanket on hand if someone gets cold is courteous.

The ambiance of your space can be set with music and essential oil diffusing as well. Bear in mind, some people are sensitive to scents so try sticking with gentler, popular scents with essential oils.

Additionally, you are going to be working pretty closely with your clients. That being said, observing personal hygiene is recommended. This includes, but is not limited to, bathing, tooth brushing, and wearing deodorant. You should be mindful of strong perfumes, soaps, and body sprays and should avoid them when working with others.

When meeting a new client for the first time, make sure to set some time aside to speak with them about Reiki, what to expect during a session, what is expected of them during a session, as well as the reason for their visit. You are going to want them to feel comfortable and relaxed. Building a trust bond between client and practitioner is important.

At this time, you can also discuss if they would like hands-on Reiki or hands-off Reiki. There are some positions, over the pubis and coccyx, where you aren't going to want to have physical contact anyway. However, some clients prefer to be touched while others don't. You'll want to respect their wishes during the treatment.

Before you touch a client, you are going to want to wash your hands with soap and water. This is for hygiene reasons, but washing the hands also helps create a clearer channel for Reiki energy.

As with your self-treatment, you are going to start at your client's head and work your way down. The provided hand positions are a rough outline of what you should be using when working on clients.

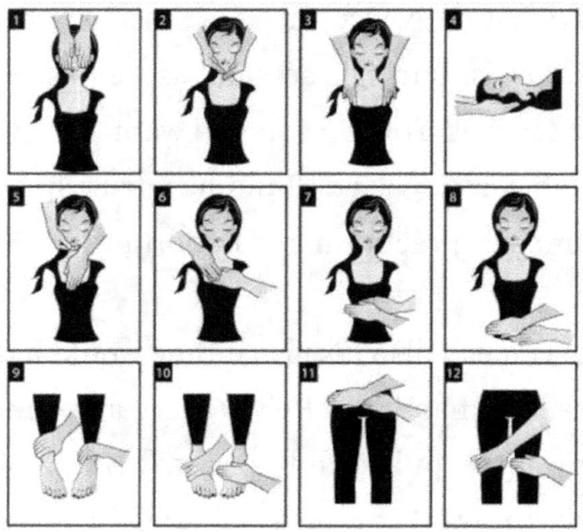

Keep in mind that even if you stick to these positions, you should be ready to listen to your intuition should it guide you in a different direction.

Your intuition can also help guide you in using Reiki symbols, crystals, and the three pillars of Reiki when working on others.

After you perform a Reiki session on a client, wash your hands again. Give them some time to get up off the table and encourage them to move slowly. After a Reiki session, it is not uncommon for clients to feel light-headed or disoriented and they may need to center themselves. In some cases, you might need to offer your clients assistance getting up off a table.

You may find some clients want to tell you everything they experience. Encourage them to do so as it can help you with their treatment plan, but don't be pushy.

Reiki treatments can be highly emotional, so having a box of tissues on hand is another good idea when performing sessions on others.

The more you work with other people, the more comfortable you will get to working with them and talking to them before and after. Any visions, ideas, emotions, or sensations you receive while working on a client is going to probably relate to them in some significant way.

While you can't interpret the meaning behind something for someone else, if you tell them and they aren't sure, you can offer a generic possibility that might give them an idea or help them determine the meaning.

For example, if you see a butterfly and they don't know the significance, offer an explanation like:

> *"Butterflies can be a symbol of transformation."*

This gives them an option to think about, but if it doesn't resonate, then they might better be able to determine how it relates.

A note on performing Reiki session for other people, unless you have other professional qualifications, Reiki practitioners cannot diagnose or prescribe. What this means is you cannot tell a Reiki client that they need to take a certain supplement, medication, get more exercise, etc. You can offer a recommendation, but no outright prescriptions.

Some good phrases to use in recommendations or suggestions are:

"I would recommend that you look into this...."

Or

"I suggest trying this out if you'd like...."

Or

"Something that has worked for me and other clients is...."

That leaves it up to the client to decide how they want to proceed with their treatment and you don't cross any legal or professional boundaries.

The same goes for diagnosing. You cannot tell a client that they have cancer or a sprained ankle, or tell them that they have pneumonia. Even if you are one hundred percent sure that is what it is, the diagnosis must come from a licensed medical professional.

You can, however, let them know there is something they might want to get looked at.

Some non-diagnostic phrases include:

"If your lungs start to feel congested, you might want to consult your doctor."

Or

"If you start to experience additional pain, getting a second opinion from a health care professional might not be a bad idea."

Or

"Next time you see your doctor, you could ask about...."

Again, this is an attempt to avoid legal entanglements and misdiagnoses. It also leaves the care in the clients' hands.

To end a Reiki session on a client, hover your hand over each of their chakras, or fluff their aura, or gently touch the bottoms of their feet for a minute. Find a comfortable method for you to help close the Reiki session for yourself and your client.

Distance Treatments

There may be times when you are asked to perform Reiki sessions on clients that are far away. You will have to be at least a Reiki Level II practitioner to perform distance Reiki as the symbol for sending Reiki across time and space is learned at Level II.

There are a few different ways to perform a distance Reiki session.

One method is to set the intention that your body is representing your client's body during the session. Then you will proceed with treatment on yourself like normal, using hand positions and intuition to guide you.

Another method for distance treatments is to use a doll or stuffed animal to represent your client. You will set the intention that the doll or stuffed animal represents your client for the session and then work through the hand positions normally.

The third method used for distance Reiki sessions is to have a picture of your client. Set the intention that the picture represents your client and then perform the session with hand symbols as the picture allows.

Distance Reiki sessions are powerful and the distance does not take away from the effectiveness. It is worth mentioning that you should never perform a session on someone unless they have asked you to perform a session or they have otherwise given you permission.

While Reiki is great and everyone can benefit from it, performing a session on someone without their permission is almost like slipping a painkiller into someone else's sandwich. They might be complaining of the pain and you want to help them feel better, but forcing them to take treatment without their consent is a major violation. The same goes for Reiki. Not everyone is ready to heal or work through the pain or accept Reiki as a treatment.

You will still want to wash your hands before and after a distance session to keep the energy channels flowing properly.

Animal Treatments

Did you know that Reiki can also be used on animals and pets?

People love pampering their pets, and Reiki, as it gains popularity, is just another way to do so!

Working with pets is going to be a little different than working with people. Partially because pets tend to have minds of their own. Generally speaking, when you perform a session on an animal, they will respond immediately to the energy. Animals are incredibly intuitive.

Reiki for animals can treat physical ailments or issues, behavioral issues, and even help pet owners.

Since pets are intuitive and energetic, sometimes, they will take on the pain for their owners. That being said, treating a pet who is exhibiting issues, as the pet heals, they will pass that along to their owner.

Some animals won't let you touch them when you are working on them. It is important to respect animals' desires. If they do allow you to touch them, they may move their body in order to get you to place your hands in a specific place.

If you are able to work hands-on, start from the head and work your way down.

During a Reiki session on an animal, they might want to get in your lap or be close to you. Reversely, they may go lie down in another room and fall asleep. However they respond, respect that. Don't follow them around or try to force hand positions on them.

If possible, perform Reiki sessions in the animals' home where they are comfortable. This will help keep them relaxed for the session.

When doing Reiki on pets and animals, they will guide the session with their own intuition. That means they will let you know when they have had enough. Maybe they will start playing, or they will resume normal activity for themselves, or whine to go outside. As your intuition develops, you'll understand the subtle hints from the animals you work on as well.

When performing a session on an animal, if they are not the only animal in the house, do not be surprised if it turns into a group session with the other pets in the house. They will sense the work you are doing and will probably want to join in especially cats.

Distance Reiki can be performed on animals as well. Having a picture or doll that you set the intention to represent your animal client the same as with a human client.

If you want to learn more about Animal Reiki, there are additional courses and resources that you can find information about animal chakras and energy systems. Having a basic understanding of their anatomy and physiology, common ailments, and the strong bond between pet and owner is a good starting point as well.

Always wash your hands thoroughly before and after working on animals. This is primarily for hygiene reasons when it comes to touching other people's pets.

When working with animals, you cannot prescribe or diagnose, unless you have additional professional qualifications. However, if something does come up that is concerning you can bring it up with the owner.

Try phrasing such as:

"You may want to ask your vet about...."

Or

"While working on your pet, I noticed...."

Since pets are essentially a part of their owners, any visions or sensations you have you may want to bring up with the owners because they might have a better idea of what the symbolism stands for.

There will be times when an animal is completely absorbing their owner's pain, trauma, or illness. If this happens, the owner may not realize it, because the pet is the one that is presenting issues.

While treating the pet does allow the energy to also flow to the owner, you might also want to gently approach the topic with the owner.

Using statements like:

"It isn't uncommon for pets to absorb the emotional and physical pains of their owners. If

You don't want to accuse or blame them. You also don't want to make them feel forced into getting a session for themselves. It also allows them to think about it and make their own informed decision.

Additional Uses for Reiki

Reiki isn't just about healing treatments and sessions with hand positions and heavy energy work. While that is a great added benefit, you, as the practitioner, have the opportunity to utilize Reiki so much more in your life!

This goes back to the concept of a Reiki lifestyle of living Reiki.

You can use Reiki as a form of attracting what you want for yourself. I know, that sounds crazy, right? Reiki to help you get what you want? Well, thinking of it in terms of energy, it isn't that crazy! We've talked about how energy can't be created nor destroyed, only transformed. So, why can't Reiki be used to transform the energy around you into something you want? Well, it can be!

There are a few different ways to implement Reiki as a tool of attraction.

One method is to Manifestation. The idea behind Manifestation is that you continue to express to the world and universe what you want, then the universe will provide it for you. Some people will speak manifestations aloud. Others will write them down on paper. Still, others might meditate around their manifestations.

How does Reiki factor into this? Well if you speak your manifestations aloud, try intoning a Reiki symbol along with your statement. This will beam Reiki energy into your manifested desires.

If you prefer writing your manifestations on paper, once they are written, use your finger to draw and intone Reiki symbols over the paper. If you are a Level I practitioner, hold the paper in the palms of your hands and intend the flow of Reiki into that paper.

When meditating for manifesting, you can include Reiki energy, symbols, or the three pillars to enhance your meditation and manifestations with Reiki.

Now, since Reiki is intuitive, if you are asking Reiki to deliver a green, fire breathing, hundred-foot dragon to your door, it probably isn't going to happen. Part of manifesting properly is coming up with realistic and attainable desires.

Additionally, if you are manifesting that a long lost love comes back to you, if they are happily married now, or if they aren't a good fit for you, the Reiki energy might find a different way to manifest your desires. That is the intuitive power of Reiki.

Reiki can be used to increase your own life force. This goes in line with self-Reiki treatments, but it isn't limited to self-Reiki.

What is life force energy? Is it your passions, your creativity, your physical energy, or your enjoyment of life? The answer to that is yes, life force energy is all of those and more.

Self-Reiki treatments can definitely help with life force energy, but there are other ways.

If you are an artist and having difficulty with creativity or ideas, try intoning an appropriate Reiki symbol on your canvas or sketchbook. You could even beam Reiki symbol or Reiki energy into the room that you do your work.

If you have trouble sleeping at night and it is making you physically exhausted, try performing a self-Reiki session while you're going to bed. This should be separate from your daily treatment because the goal of this session is specifically to put you to sleep.

Maybe you'll just hold your hands on your head or over your heart. Perhaps, you will intone a Reiki symbol into your pillow. Using Reiki to help relax you into a peaceful sleep can definitely improve your physical energy.

That being said, maybe you are trying to cut caffeine out of your diet and it is making you sluggish. Well, Reiki is a great tool for helping with addictions.

Every time you want a cup of coffee or some soda, intone the appropriate Reiki symbol for yourself or do a quick 5-minute session with a hand position on your head to help boost your alertness and mental energy.

Reiki can even be infused into food to help you better absorb nutrients and balance out potentially harmful chemicals. Holding your plate or bowl and performing a quick Reiki session, or using symbols on your food is a great way to infuse food with Reiki. What better way to nurture your life energy than with food!?

Another beneficial use for Reiki outside of treatments is mediation or transforming negative situations or problems.

If you and a friend, spouse, or family member got into an argument, try beaming Reiki energy directly into the time and space of the argument. When you decide to reconcile and discuss what happened, send Reiki energy to the time and place of the conversation.

You can also beam Reiki energy into the room that the discussion is going to take place in. This will help create a peaceful and relaxed environment. It will also promote positivity.

If you would like to use Reiki directly during a conflict, if emotions are high or heavy, take a moment to channel Reiki into yourself. You may find clarity in the argument. You may find a solution that presents itself for the situation, or you could simply diffuse the situation so that it can be discussed rationally.

That being said, since Reiki can be sent over time and space, you can also use Reiki to transform past negative events and resolve past problems that may still be lingering.

Going even further than that, Reiki can be sent across generational barriers. Generational traumas can be passed down for years without being addressed. Sending Reiki back through time to treat a problem that began, a generation trauma can provide relief in the present or future.

Past lives can have negative experiences that leave a lingering trauma in our current lives. Reiki energy can be used to heal and transform past life trauma and pain as well which will provide balance in the present or future.

The uses for Reiki are innumerable in both sessions and in everyday life. The more you play around with using Reiki in your life, the more uses you will find for it.

Chapter Four: Chakras, Auras, and Energy Shields

Energetic anatomy, subtle bodies, or energy systems are all terms for the same concept. The body has various energy fields and energy sources that contribute to overall health and wellness. Two of the better-known systems are the aura system and the chakra system.

Just like the rest of the body, these systems need attention and maintenance to keep flowing. These are the systems that contribute to the personal energy fields and frequencies that everyone gives off.

Chakras

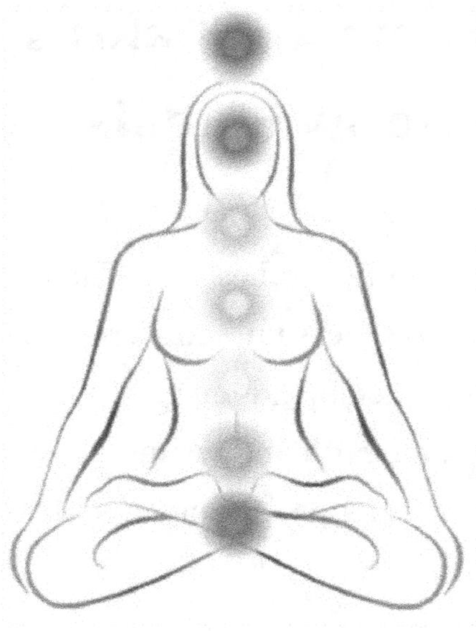

The chakra system is comprised of seven main chakras that are energetic centers in the body. They sit along the spine and are cone-shaped extending out from the spine in the front and the back of the body.

The seven main chakras are the Crown Chakra, Third Eye Chakra, Throat Chakra, Heart Chakra, Solar Plexus Chakra, Sacral Chakra, and the Root Chakra.

Each chakra has different associations. These associations contribute to physical, emotional, and mental health.

Chakras are a huge source of energy flow in the body. If one chakra is blocked, this can restrict the energy flow to Chakras below it on the spin. If a chakra is overactive, that can create overactivity in the chakras below it on the spine as well.

Energy flow in the bodies and chakras should be balanced and steady. Depending on if a chakra is blocked or overactive, different symptoms can arise. These symptoms can be physical, emotional, or mental. However, since Reiki is intuitive and goes where it is needed, as the Practitioner, you do not need to know if a chakra is blocked or overactive.

Crystals can be great when working with Reiki and chakras as well. Most crystals have a chakra association based on their color because all chakras have a color association as well.

When performing Reiki session on yourself or others, starting or ending the session by touching each of the seven chakras can help ensure a complete balancing of the energy. Plus, to some clients, it feels nice to have their chakras stimulated.

<u>Crown Chakra:</u>
The Crown Chakra is set close to the top of the brain. Its cone point is at the head and it opens upwards towards the sky. This chakra is associated with the pineal gland and the emotional association is bliss.

When imbalanced, you can feel a limited connection with the divine or spirit. The body's inner wisdom is hard to access, and it leads to mental imbalances. This can manifest in headaches, nightmares, and vision or eye problems.

When properly balanced, you experience the wisdom of the self and the universe. You are self-aware and have self-realization.

The color associated with the crown chakra is violet or light purple. Some common crystals that can help balance the crown chakra include amethyst and clear quartz.

Third Eye Chakra

This chakra is located between the eyes on the forehead in the front of the body and at the base of the occiput on the back of the body. It is associated with the pituitary gland. Emotional associations include fear and imagination.

When imbalanced, the third eye chakra leads to poor vision, close-mindedness, headaches, mental and hormonal issues, and sleep issues. These can also manifest as depression, anguish, and mental turmoil.

When properly balanced, the third eye chakra promotes creativity, healthy intuition, strong memory, manifestation, and balanced hormones.

The Third Eye Chakra is represented by the color indigo or dark blue. A common crystal associated with the third eye chakra is lapis lazuli.

<u>Throat Chakra</u>

The Throat Chakra is located at the base of the throat in the front and the base of the neck in the back. It is associated with the larynx, vocal cords, thyroid, and expression. An expression can be verbal and emotional.

When imbalanced, the throat chakra affects communication. People can be overly talkative of non-communicative. Thyroid issues can present with an imbalanced throat chakra as well as metabolic and hormonal conditions. Coughing and wheezing are also related to the throat chakra. Imbalances can lead to a stiff neck, sore throat, and hearing problems.

When balanced, the throat chakra leads to strong communication, expression of personal truth, and the maintaining of healthy weight.

The throat chakra is blue in color. Crystals that work to balance the throat chakra include blue lace agate and celestite.

<u>Heart Chakra</u>

The heart chakra is located in the center of the sternum on the front and between the base of the shoulder blades on the back. The heart chakra is associated with the heart organ as well as the heart center which is behind the physical heart. It is also related to the thymus gland. Emotional associations include love and joy.

When imbalanced, the heart chakra creates a problem in which the person does not accept love. It can create problems in relationships, holding grudges, lung and heart issues, and immune system imbalances. There can also be a lack of self-confidence, fear, and self-destructive tendencies.

When the heart chakra is balanced it opens up to the ability to give and receive love. The immune system is healthy and balanced. Relationships are healthy and balanced, as well as promoting compassion, peace, and harmony.

The heart chakra is associated with the color green. There is an upper heart chakra, that is a sub chakra, which is associated with the color pink. Both colors are acceptable to work with for the heart chakra. Common crystals to use on the heart chakra include emerald, malachite, and rose quartz.

Solar Plexus Chakra

The solar plexus chakra is located an inch or two above the navel in the front and a couple of inches above the sacrum on the back. The organs associated with the solar plexus chakra include the liver, spleen, gallbladder, pancreas, and stomach. Emotions connected to the solar plexus chakra are anger and having a sense of purpose. This is also where the inner child resides.

An imbalanced solar plexus leads to confusion about your role in the world. Feelings of rejection and issues with the associated organs. It can also lead to extreme introversion or extroversion. It can also present as poor decision-making, nervous system and immune system issues, and low vitality.

When the solar plexus chakra is balanced, it promotes healthy digestion in matters of both food and life experiences. It also creates a feeling of personal power and confidence.

This chakra is the color yellow. A couple of crystals that resonate with the solar plexus chakra are citrine and tiger's eye.

<u>Sacral Chakra</u>

Located an inch or two below the navel on the front and located in the center of the sacrum in the back, the sacral chakra is connected to reproductive organs and kidneys. It is associated with emotions of joy and desire.

If the sacral chakra becomes imbalanced, it can present as over-sexuality or low libido. There can be imbalances around creativity, possessiveness, and jealousy. The immune system can have problems. It also leads to low self-esteem. Feelings of boredom, over seriousness, resentment, disdain, and inability to let go of the past. Bladder and urinary issues can develop.

When the sacral chakra is balanced, this leads to high self-esteem, healthy sexuality, healthy creativity, as well as joy and pleasure.

The sacral chakra is depicted as orange in color. Some crystals that work well with the sacral chakra include amber and red jasper.

Root Chakra

Located at the base of the spine at the coccyx. This chakra has its point at the base of the spine and points down towards the feet. It is associated with the kidneys and adrenal glands. Emotional correspondences are fear and passion.

The root chakra is the center of survival and our personal foundation and strength. When imbalanced, this leads to insecurity, being spaced out, and fatigue. It can present as fear around survival. Imbalances can be in the form of obesity, constipation, any problems associated with the feet, legs, blood, and bones. Hemorrhoids are also associated with the blocked root chakra.

When the root chakra is probably balanced, it creates a feeling of being grounded. It promotes motivation and feeling comfortable in the physical world.

The root chakra is red. Crystals associated with the root chakra include garnet, ruby, obsidian, and smoky quartz.

Since the root and sacral chakra are more intimately placed on the body, placing your hand directly on the body to touch them is not a good idea, but you can still hover your hands over the position.

As you work with your clients and talk to them about symptoms and feelings, you will start to make associations with specific chakras and blockages or overactivity. This is where crystals can become useful in Reiki treatments to target specific chakras with the crystals.

Aura

The aura is an energy field that exists around the entire body. If you've ever heard the term 'personal bubble,' that is essentially what the aura is.

People who extend their auras out away from their bodies expand their personal bubble to keep everyone else at a distance. People who keep their aura closer to their bodies allow other people to get much closer to them. This is physical proximity. That energetic field does send out a frequency. Even if it is completely unconscious, we expand and contract our auras regularly, depending on the situations we find ourselves in.

Auras can have colors that indicate an energetic frequency. If you are unfamiliar with auras, you should start developing your ability to see auras. You can do this by getting yourself comfortable and taking several deep breaths.

Inhale to the count of four and exhale to the count of eight. Once your mind starts to relax, look at another person or at an animal. You might want to avoid practicing on strangers so it doesn't look like you are staring.

Stop focusing your eyes on their physical body and start looking at the space around the outline of their body. Try to stare at that space around their outline, and you should start to be able to see their aura. There are other methods of learning how to see auras, so find one that works for you.

The basic makeup of the aura is in seven auric layers around the body. Each layer corresponds to a chakra and has other associations.

The first auric layer is about 1-2 inches from the body and it is associated with the root chakra.

The second auric layer is 3-4 inches away from the body and connects to the sacral chakra.

The third layer of the aura is associated with the solar plexus chakra and it is about 5-6 inches away from the body.

The fourth layer is connected to the heart chakra. This is a very important aura layer when it comes to emotions and energy. It sits between 7-8 inches from the body.

The fifth layer of the aura is associated with the throat chakra. This is also the color layer of the chakra. Pastel colors are usually healthy and balanced. The fifth layer sits about 9-10 inches from the body.

The sixth auric layer is 11-12 inches from the body and is connected with the third eye chakra and is silver in color. It is an energy shield for the body. It can get cracked, and Reiki can help heal those cracks.

The seventh auric layer is about 13-14 inches away from the body. It resonates with the crown chakra, connecting to the universe and wisdom. This aura is made up of white or silver energy beads. They can become dingy or off-color over time and Reiki and crystals can be used to revitalize them.

The aura is kind of the natural defense that the body has for unwanted energies. It is very important to take care of the aura and keep it healthy for this reason.

Your aura is going to also be the truest expression of your own energy frequency. The aura's color can change depending on what frequency you are operating on, energetically.

Some different techniques for cleansing the aura include guided meditations, crystal work, Reiki, and non-guided meditation with an intention to clear the aura.

Clear quartz is a fantastic crystal for aura clearing as it is considered a 'heal-all' crystal that can work with any kind of ailment or energy. During your Reiki studies, you may learn more advanced techniques for using both Reiki and crystals to clear the individual aura layers. This work can get deep but is so beneficial.

Take some time to get to know your own chakras and your own aura. Understanding them within yourself can help you understand them in other people. More importantly, it can help you understand yourself and help you feel connected to yourself.

The body is a fine-tuned machine, like a car. It requires maintenance, like oil changes, air in the tires, car washes, engine tune-ups, etc. The body is similar. But you don't ignore the maintenance requirements of your car just because you can't see the oil tank, so why ignore the needs of your unseen energy systems?

Energy Shields

When performing energy work on other people, it is important to be aware of the fact that you become vulnerable. Your clients are going to be releasing a lot of energy and it is going to be shifting, which will residually impact you.

Now, since Reiki is channeled through you in only one direction, you won't absorb energy back through your client because of Reiki. What this means is that you channel the energy from the universe into your body and then transfer it into your client. Your client doesn't transfer anything back, because it is a one-way flow.

That being said, as your client releases energy and blockages, that energy doesn't just disappear. Remember, energy cannot be created or destroyed, just transformed.

So, what happens to it? A lot of times, that energy lingers in the space where you perform Reiki. Sometimes, it will latch on to an object or person. This is how it can residually latch on to you.

When doing energy work, you are going to want to take measures to protect yourself from residual energy. You don't want to accidentally pick up something that starts to have a negative impact on your life. Especially if it goes unnoticed, it can fester and create bigger problems.

Additionally, when working on clients, it is incredibly easy to get 'sucked in' to their energy field. This isn't necessarily a bad thing, depending on the work you are doing. However, it is a good practice to keep your energy fields separated.

Energy shielding is the term used to describe protecting yourself, or shielding yourself, from the residual energies of other people.

You'll have to play around with energy shielding to find the best method for yourself. A common energy shielding technique is to imagine yourself with a protective bubble around you that deflects any unwanted energy from you.

You can replace the bubble with a silver wall or another protective color that you resonate with.

A couple of other methods are in terms of ensuring you are grounded so you don't absorb the wrong energies or get sucked into someone else's energies. Having a strong visualization of tree roots around your legs and ankles can help keep you firmly grounded.

Imagining yourself as a rock in a stream is a good method, too. If you are the rock, then the energy is the water and it flows around you, but it doesn't affect you.

Energy shielding is the best way to hold your own space and prevent yourself from becoming encumbered by unwanted energies.

Those energies are still being released into space you are practicing Reiki in, you are also going to want to make sure space is held safely.

Before performing a session, you can beam Reiki symbols into the room with the intention of holding a safe and clear space. This will ensure a balanced environment, but also help create a relaxed feeling for the client. Your room should feel comfortable as they enter into it.

Before you perform a Reiki session, you can use intention combined with Reiki power to set a safe and clear space as well. Whether you speak the intention aloud or just visualize it strongly in your mind, that will set the ground for the safe space.

Also, intoning Reiki symbols into the table or chair your client will be on can help keep them clear and the space around them clear.

Cleaning with Reiki

While taking preemptive measures is important, sometimes, it is necessary to do additional clearings of space and tools after a session. Reiki is a powerful cleansing energy as well.

If you decide to use crystals in your Reiki sessions, it is important to cleanse them regularly. Crystals are highly absorptive, especially when it comes to energy. While they can harmlessly absorb energy from someone, that means they then store the energy. You wouldn't want to use a crystal storing someone else's energy to try and clear a different client.

First of all, crystals can get full. They are like hard drives. Too much information and they become less effective. Second of all, if that energy is just being stored, it isn't being transmuted in the universe to become something positive. While that won't affect your or the client directly, it is a service to the universe as a whole to allow the energy to be transmuted.

Reiki energy can be used to clear crystals. This can be done by holding a crystal in your palm and calling on the flow of Reiki energy. You will want to continue the energetic flow until your intuition tells you the crystal is clear.

If you are Attuned to Level II Reiki, you can intone and draw Reiki symbols on the crystals to clear them.

Other crystal cleansing methods include running them under cool water (make sure the crystal won't dissolve in water as some do), setting out in moonlight or sunlight (make sure the crystal isn't damaged by direct sunlight as some are), submerging in a dish of rock salt, or passing through the smoke of a smudge stick or incense.

You will also want to use Reiki to clear yourself and your practice space. Ideally done before and after every session, even with your energy shielding, this will keep promoting balance and preventing anything from slipping through the cracks.

Reiki symbols are great to put on windows and doorways. This helps keep energy out of the room and can create a physical difference in energy for people passing through the door.

You can clear yourself with Reiki before and after sessions with a quick 5-minute self-treatment with only a couple hand positions. You can also use Reiki symbols drawn on yourself to clear your own body and energy bodies before and after sessions.

If you end up having a busy schedule and don't have time to clear yourself in between sessions, it is imperative that you do a thorough cleaning at the beginning of your day and at the end of your day. Ideally, on yourself and space you work in.

Energetic anatomy is just as vital to health as physical anatomy. Many modern medicines have unfortunately turned away from the understanding and knowledge of energies and how they impact the body. As a Reiki practitioner, this puts you in a somewhat unique position to help educate your clients, friends, and family (if they are interested) in how to maintain their energetic health.

When it comes to using Reiki for clearing spaces, people, objects, and yourself, there aren't necessarily the right and wrong ways. The methods provided in this book are commonly used to give you a starting point. You will find what methods you prefer and what methods resonate with you as you continue to practice.

Even if you aren't performing Reiki on other people, using Reiki to clear yourself and your home is another practical application of this energy work.

Chapter Five: Reiki Lifestyle

There are many ways to incorporate Reiki into your lifestyle. Daily treatments on yourself are just a part of living Reiki and using it to guide you through your day. Whether it is diet, exercise, work, parenting, relationships, etc., Reiki can guide you and raise the vibration of your life.

Reiki and Food

We've touched on using Reiki with food, but now, it will be covered in a little more detail. When it comes to food, the quality of food you are eating is going to be very important. It is important for personal health, but it is also important for the cleanliness of the body.

As a Reiki practitioner, you are going to be channeling pure universal energy through you. As a conduit, you are going to want to remain healthy. If you are able to regularly eat clean foods, such as organic and unprocessed foods, you will remain a clearer channel for Reiki.

The clearer your body is the more sensitive your intuition and energy will become to the energy of your clients. This can make you a more effective energy worker.

Changing your eating habits or changing the kind of food you keep in your kitchen is going to be beneficial as you practice and learn Reiki.

It is so easy to come across unhealthy foods, overly processed foods, and mass-produced foods that are full of hormones, preservatives, and potentially harmful chemicals. In our society, those foods seem to be more easily accessible. Whether you are eating conventional foods or organic foods, including Reiki is a good way to get the most out of your food.

Being committed to a cleaner and healthier eating may not be easy, but if you are serious about being a Reiki practitioner, be more conscious about the foods and drinks that you are putting in your body.

That being said, Reiki energy can be used to raise the vibration of the food you eat. You can use these techniques on organic and conventional foods.

Using Reiki with your food is going to start when you are shopping for groceries. Whether at a Farmer's market, grocery store, natural food store, or supermarket, you can default to your intuition to find specific food items that will serve your higher good.

Call on Reiki energies as you are shopping with the intention of connecting with the food you want to buy.

Once the food is at home and in your kitchen, you can use either Reiki symbols, or a little Reiki energy to clear each food item as you put them away. This will help remove any residual energies the food items picked up from where they were grown, the store they were in, and on their travels to your home.

When preparing food to eat, using the Reiki distance symbol, or just a strong intent with Reiki energy can help you connect with the source of your food, i.e. the farm it was grown on, the animal, or plant it came from.

Having that deeper connection with the energy of the source of your food is going to help imbue each meal with a deeper energetic connection. When you connect with your food energetically, you'll absorb more of the nutrients, clear away potentially harmful energies and toxins, but also deepen your own connection to life and energy.

Being a Reiki practitioner, having that strong connection to life and the source of energy is going to help you grow and progress as a healer.

Once a meal is prepared, use Reiki symbols or Reiki energy on the bowl or plate that you are eating from. Then serve yourself and use more Reiki energy over the entire meal. Also, charge your drinks with Reiki energy.

On a more serious note, if you are struggling with an eating disorder, Reiki can be beneficial in helping recover from that.

If eating is difficult for you in one way or another, trying performing Reiki on yourself before eating. Doing a quick session on yourself before a meal, or use Reiki symbols can help with the eating disorder or problems around eating.

Many people develop issues with eating, whether it is emotional eating or under eating, there are a lot of different manifestations of eating disorders. Some people associate food with negative experiences or abuse and it makes eating an uncomfortable experience.

This should never be the case! Eating should always be enjoyable. So, even if the act of eating is the problem and not the food itself, using Reiki on yourself and the food you are eating can help to overcome those disorders and those inhibitors.

Another option is to send Reiki to the time and place that you are going to be eating. That way once the meal begins, you can ease in with the Reiki energy guiding you.

You'll get the feel for how to use Reiki with your food. Food is our primary nourishment, so supplying that source of nourishment with the benefit of Reiki just strengthens our own nourishment and life force.

Working with energy is, in many ways, about connecting. Connecting to yourself, connecting to your spirit, and connecting to the universe and the energies of others. Bringing that connection into different aspects of your life, such as food and eating, is going to continue to bring your life fulfillment and satisfaction.

Reiki and Exercise

Movement is vital to life. Not only is movement required to keep our lymphatic system working, but movement prevents joint stiffness, muscle problems, and even bone problems.

Many individuals who don't exercise gain weight, lose feeling in extremities due to loss of circulation, have chronic pain from too much pressure being put on certain body parts while sitting or standing in the same positions, or in more severe cases, develop atrophied muscles.

Now, these are pretty extreme. It takes years of excessive not exercising to produce such results. However, movement and exercise are still vital.

In a lot of societies right now, movement and exercise aren't exactly encouraged. The majority of jobs are desk-based that require people to sit pretty much in a stationary position for 8 to 10 hours.

So much of our culture is based around computers, social media, phones, and even video games that after a day of work, or on days off, people lean more towards relaxing on the couch or at a desk rather than going out for physical activity.

Then there is the problem that many people have had where they had a negative experience with exercise. Whether it is because they were always picked last for sports on the playground, or they fell on a treadmill or were made fun of for their weight while out walking or running, a lot of people have had negative experiences with exercise.

So how can Reiki help?

Honestly, Reiki can help you be whoever you want to be!

If you have trouble exercising or are trying to motivate yourself to exercise more, put your workout clothes on and then give yourself a quick 10-minute treatment. After that, do some stretching, and then give yourself another ten-minute treatment. You can also use Reiki symbols as needed.

The distance symbol HSZSN that you learn in Level II Reiki is monumental in helping heal past traumas, insecurities, and bad experiences. If you use it while you are wearing your workout clothes, or before or after a light workout, it can help to heal those past experiences.

You can also use Reiki in manifesting motivation to exercise. Maybe you just feel too tired to exercise or have no motivation to actually do it! So write down your exercise goals on a piece of paper. Try to make them realistic. Maybe start with shorter-term goals in the beginning. Use Reiki symbols on the paper, or hold the paper in your hands and call for Reiki energy.

Keep that paper in your pocket anytime you do anything physical, whether it is a simple walk or a more rigorous workout routine.

You might not have any trouble getting yourself to exercise, but seeking to reach a specific goal with exercise, such as weight loss. Reiki energy and Reiki symbols can help to promote such a goal.

If weight loss is your goal for workouts, balancing symbol SHK that you learn in Level II Reiki is also a great symbol to promote weight loss. Use the symbol specifically on the areas of the body that you would like to lose weight from before you start your workout routine.

If you aren't Attuned to Level II, hold your hands over a specific area of the body you would like to lose weight from and let Reiki flow there before you start a workout.

Another way to incorporate Reiki into exercise to make the most of it is, if you already have a workout routine, trying having Reiki energy flow through the entire workout. Almost like a combo workout and self-treatment session.

This can be done for rigorous workouts or for a simple and easy walk. Either way, intending that you receive Reiki for the duration of the workout or exercise will really take it to the next level.

You might lose weight faster, get toned muscles faster, find your endurance increasing, having more motivation to exercise, or just simply feeling more connected to your own body and skin.

Getting into a good exercise routine and making healthy habits out of exercise is going to take a little time. Reiki can help motivate you and help you reach your exercise goals. It can also help you overcome any adversities you have in regards to exercise.

Reiki and Water

Water and hydration are such an important part of the human existence, that it deserves additional attention away from food.

There are plenty of studies to show how water molecules are impacted by energy vibes. It was touched on previously how positive words, thoughts, and feelings alter the molecular structure of water the same way negative thoughts, words, and feelings do.

Everyone should be drinking water daily. More than that, we use water to wash our hands, wash our dishes, bath our bodies, water our plants, etc. There are endless uses for water around the house.

Reiki energy can be used to improve water quality and give it healing, balancing power. With a glass of water that you intone a Reiki symbol into or channel Reiki energy into, the taste of the water changes. Even if ever so subtly.

Using Reiki energy on the water meant for your plants and gardens can help promote healthy and abundant plant growth.

Washing your hands in Reiki treated water will help keep your hands a pure and clean channel for healing yourself and clients.

Start treating the water that you drink, water plants with, and wash your hands with Reiki energy. You might be pleasantly surprised in the differences you start to notice.

Reiki can be used to turn water into a healing elixir. By drinking Reiki treated water, those treated molecules can change the energy vibration of the rest of the water molecules in your body!

The origin of life is in water, from the very oceans of our planet. This makes water a powerful source of life energy. Even if it is coming from a tap, that water is still connected back to the source. Therefore, using Reiki on the water is going to increase your connection to life energy and improve your overall vibration.

Reiki Blessings

You can also start to use Reiki in blessings. Blessings don't have to be major or formal, but add a little Reiki to them and start to see how the environment around you improves.

If you are a plant owner or gardener, use Reiki to bless seeds or potted plants by channeling Reiki energy into the seeds as you hold them, or by putting your hands on either side of a plant pot. You can also use Reiki symbols on seeds and pots.

Or you can bless an entire garden with Reiki. If you are a first-time gardener or starting something new, like a vegetable garden, offering some Reiki energy can help ensure healthy plant growth.

If you are moving into a new house or apartment, blessing each room with Reiki before moving in can ensure a happy stay in the home. Channel energy directly into the room, or use Reiki symbols to beam the energy into the rooms. If you are buying a house or moving into an apartment with a romantic partner for the first time, use Reiki to bless the space for harmonious coexistence.

Maybe you have a job interview coming up and want to ensure that it goes smoothly. Send Reiki to the time and place of the interview, blessing it with balancing energy and success. The distance symbol learned in Level II Reiki is the best method for sending Reiki energy through time and space.

Small Reiki blessings can be used in all kinds of scenarios throughout the day. Getting in the habit of using Reiki energy during your daily activities will literally transform the environment around you. The balancing energy will go where it needs to and as you work on yourself too, you will start to attract the types of things into your life that you resonate with.

So, working on yourself while adding small Reiki blessings into your own world, you start to create the world that you truly want for yourself. The idea of blessings may seem odd or like a religious concept.

In this case, blessings are simply adding positive or balanced energy to situations or aspects of your life. Reiki has innumerable uses when it is applied to seemingly menial daily activities and tasks.

The more you practice, the more it will become a habit for you to call on Reiki every day. This is how you start truly living Reiki.

Reiki and the World

Using Reiki to change your own environment and the direct world around you is great for your personal life and personal abundance and health. However, since Reiki can be sent across time and space, sometimes, using it on a larger scale can be helpful.

For example, if there is a natural disaster in part of the world, setting aside time to send Reiki energy to that area of the world and to the relief efforts can lend a helping hand. It can also improve the mood and overall conditions of life in areas that have been harmed by natural disasters.

A single Reiki practitioner won't have the power to completely alter the course of an entire natural disaster relief effort. However, every little bit helps, and if other Reiki practitioners are pitching in, which they should be, then more energy will keep getting sent to that area.

Reiki energy can be sent into specific situations as well. Consider political situations or areas of conflict and war in the world. By sending Reiki energy into those situations, the balancing and healing process begins. While one practitioner may not be able to change an entire political situation or end a war, as long as practitioners are sending out the healing energy into these situations, change will happen. Change in the form of balance and healing.

Maybe there is an area of the world that is suffering from a drought or crop blight. While in our modern society that might not seem like such a big deal, but droughts and blights and other types of famines can and do still occur. Their impact may be localized, but it is still an impact.

Reiki energy can be used to try and relieve the impact of such blights. Reiki can help rebalance the environment to bring rain. It can rebalance soil for nutrients. Reiki can also provide balance to an ecosystem to prevent an overpopulation of crop pests.

Most Reiki practitioners who are committed to living the Reiki lifestyle and being Reiki healers will take notice of global unrest, whether it be natural or human-based, and lend Reiki energy as needed.

Healers tend to be community-oriented. If there is a disruption in your community, offering Reiki energy can help a situation. This could be as simple as a water main break or more serious in the event of a missing child. Even from a distance, providing Reiki energy can promote a resolution or solution. In the least, it can provide balance, clarity, and relax tensions.

In a closer to a home setting, say you have a tree in your yard that is in bad health or diseased. Supplying that tree with Reiki energy can help heal the wound or disease and bring it back into a healthy state.

Reiki energy is a powerful force. It exists through the entire universe. While it is primarily used for treating yourself and other people with healing sessions, Reiki isn't limited to just treatments.

In everyday life, Reiki can be used in food, to help with exercise, and to make healing elixirs. Reiki can be used to help global situations like natural disasters, wars, and political unrest. It can work in communities to solve smaller problems and even in your physical environment. You can also include Reiki in everyday tasks and activities to change the very frequency of the world you live in!

The uses for Reiki are innumerable. To start living the Reiki lifestyle, just take a moment to think of all the times and situations in any given day that you could add some Reiki energy in order to improve that task.

Reiki can be used on people, animals, inanimate objects, and plants. Reiki can be used on manmade and natural objects. Reiki energy can be sent through time and space and to specific situations.

The more you incorporate Reiki into your everyday life, the better you will feel. The more at home you will feel in your own environment. This will lead to a more balanced and satisfactory life.

Chapter Six: Reiki and Meditation

Meditation is a common practice in Reiki. Many holistic healers and practitioners do include meditation of some kind in their lives. Whether they are yoga instructors, massage therapists, Reiki practitioners, or individuals that are committed to a full body, mind, and spirit wellness will use meditation regularly.

There are two basic forms of meditation. The first is to completely clear your mind of all thoughts. The second type of meditation is to focus on a specific question, concern, or situation.

With Reiki meditation, the focus is on Reiki energy rather than any other subject. During a Reiki meditation, you focus on the universal energy as it is within you, around you, and within everything around you. You want to feel connected to that energy to create a feeling of tranquility, connection, and peace.

Your body will feel revitalized and full of life energy. It is a very rejuvenating type of meditation.

When you meditate, it is recommended that you find a quiet place where you won't be disturbed. You'll want to set a relaxing atmosphere. Set the lights low, light some candles, maybe burn some incense or diffuse herbal oils. If music helps you relax, play a soothing soundtrack.

You can sit or lie down for meditation, but if you are prone to falling asleep, sitting up may be the best idea. While it isn't bad to fall asleep during meditation, the goal is to keep a certain focus and connection with the Reiki energy which won't be as strong if you fall asleep.

To start relaxing your mind, breathe in through your nose to the count of four and then breathe out through your mouth to the count of eight.

After a few of these deep breaths, you'll want to start focusing on Reiki energy. Start with the energy within yourself, and as you connect to it, feel it expand outward into the universe and into the space and objects around you. You should feel the energy moving through you and around you.

Keep your focus on that energy for as long as you want to, or as long as you feel called to. If you want to meditate for a certain amount of time, set some kind of timer with a gentle call back sound like a soft bell or going to let you when you should end the meditation.

Meditation can take practice. If you are unfamiliar with meditation or new to meditation, you might have to work your way up to longer meditation times. Starting with just five minutes is fairly standard.

In the beginning, it is easy to get distracted by thoughts and sounds in the room around you, like the heat coming on, the sound of a branch on the window, or thoughts of your day. Over time, with practice, these distractions won't be as prominent.

However, there are some techniques to help you stay in that meditative mindset. One method to try is when you begin to meditate, set the tip of your tongue to the top of your mouth. If your mind starts to wander, your tongue will fall from the roof of your mouth. Any time you notice this, bring your tongue back to the roof of your mouth and refocus on your meditation.

The tongue trick is somewhat similar to the Gassho finger technique in which you press your middle fingers together if you begin to experience thoughts that pull you away from your meditation. Starting a meditation with the Gassho technique can also help your mind focus when you move into a Reiki meditation.

There is a somewhat standard 21-day Reiki meditation program that can help you learn more about Reiki and also help you develop your meditation skills. It is broken down into different segments to cover the 21 days. These 21 days are also symbolic of the time that Dr. Usui spent on top of a mountain in study to reach enlightenment.

Day 1-7

Begin each mediation with the thought of a question. Start by either drawing the CKR power symbol or by calling on the flow of Reiki energy. Breathing the symbol or energy directly into your Solar Plexus chakra and hold the pure essence of Reiki there. When you exhale, allow the energy to touch and enter every cell in your body. Expand this penetration into your mental body and energetic body. Have that Reiki energy touch every part of your physical and energetic self.

For 5 to 15 minutes, sit with this power flowing through you. Hold it within you and keep it circulating to every cell in your body and energetic body. If your mind wanders, intone the CKR symbol again, or re-channel the Reiki energy into yourself.

When you have finished, acknowledge that the Reiki energy is fully within you and it will remain in you for the entire day. If you care to, make notes on anything you felt or experienced during this mediation.

Day 8-14

Begin these sessions with an intention or question as before. This time, you are going to use the SHK symbol or channel dire Reiki energy into your heart chakra. Breathe either the symbol or Reiki directly into your heart chakra and let it fill that chakra. Upon exhaling, allow the energy of that symbol or the Reiki energy to flow into every corner of your being. Let it touch every cell and atom of your physical and energetic body. Imagine any unhealthy thought patterns or emotions that you may be experiencing and envision them being remade into healthy thoughts and emotions.

Sit with this energy flow for 5 to 15 minutes. If your mind wanders at all, intone the symbol again or call more Reiki energy into yourself. When you complete your meditation, acknowledge that you are full of Reiki and full of love and that you will carry it with you through your day. Make any notes on your experiences if you wish.

Day 15-21

You will want to start these mediations with a question or intention like before. This time, you are going to intone the HSZSN symbol, or simply call Reiki energy into the crown chakra. Breathe the symbol or Reiki energy into your crown chakra and then down your spine into each of the other six main chakras.

Pull the energy through the chakras and into your limbs and extremities all the way to your fingertips and toe tips. As you exhale, let that energy disperse through every piece of your physical and energetic body.

Imagine the symbol you drew or the Reiki energy you called, forming a bright light bridge that extends through time and space. Use this bridge to send Reiki back in time and forward in time to permeate every layer of your consciousness from the beginning and going forward. Allow it to enter the different dimensions of your being.

Come back to the present moment and sit with that energy flow for 5 to 15 minutes. If your mind wanders, call yourself back with that symbol again or by channeling more Reiki energy.

Once you finish this meditation, acknowledge that the timeless power of Reiki energy and its healing qualities are being held within you and you are connected to Reiki. That it will be with you throughout the day. If you'd like, take the time to make notes on any experiences that you had or felt while meditating.

Reiki can be used in congruence with meditation in other ways as well. It isn't just about connecting yourself deeper to that universal energy.

We already discussed how Reiki and meditation work together in the Three Pillars of Reiki and the Five Principles of Reiki. Any form of Reiki mediation you decide to use or practice can be combined with those pillars and with the principles of Reiki.

Reiki meditation can also be used for cleansing and clearing the body of any unwanted or negative energies.

To cleanse your body with meditation, sit or lie down comfortably. You'll want to set a relaxing atmosphere just like with any other meditation.

Start breathing deeply, in through the nose and out through the mouth. In to the count of four and out to the count of eight. Your mind will begin to relax and feel open. Here, you will begin to channel Reiki energy.

Breathe the Reiki energy down through your crown chakra. Keep breathing it down into your third eye chakra and let it release from the front and back points of the third eye. Again, breathe Reiki energy down through the crown and into the throat chakra, releasing it out the front and back of the chakra.

Continue to breathe Reiki through the crown and down to the heart chakra, releasing it out the front and back of the chakra. Bring Reiki down through the crown and into the solar plexus chakra, releasing it out the front and back. Repeat this process for the sacral chakra as well.

Take another deep breath, breathing Reiki through your crown and down into the root chakra. Release this energy out the base of your spine and down past your feet.

Next, breathing Reiki energy up your spine, completely clearing your spine as you go and then up and out the crown chakra.

Once the chakras and spine have been cleared, focus on clean, healthy energy flow through your body and sit with that flow for as long as you would like.

This meditation can be as long or short as you want. In fact, the chakra and spine clearing portion can be performed in only a couple minutes if you are well practiced with it. This means that throughout your day if you are feeling stressed or overwhelmed, do a quick Reiki chakra clearing meditation to help cleanse your body and mind and then get back to your day.

Meditation is a useful tool for personal growth. It is also great for connecting with yourself on more than just the physical level. Meditation can provide clarity and contribute greatly to emotional health as well as physical health.

With the combination of Reiki, meditation reaches an entirely new level of benefit and it can bring you to a higher level of your own Reiki journey as a practitioner.

Going beyond meditation, Reiki also coincides with other spiritual practices and energies. Kundalini is a Hindu concept of divine energy that is located at the base of the spine. It is generally described as a sleeping force. It is potential energy that is dormant in the human body. It is part of the energetic anatomy of the body, along with chakras and auras.

Kundalini is said to be the feminine, evolutionary, and creative force of infinite wisdom. Through yoga, meditation, and Reiki, Kundalini can be awoken within the body.

What is the point of a Kundalini awakening?

Primarily, it is for self-realization. With self-realization comes the release of ego and the connection to the divine forces, such as universal energy.

Once a Kundalini awakening has occurred, it is accompanied by other intense feelings of bliss, oneness, and sometimes, can even create a mystical experience as Kundalini powerfully purifies the body.

A true Kundalini awakening can be powerful and intense, so you don't want to force an awakening, however, with the use of Reiki, you can begin the process of a Kundalini awakening and when the time is right, this powerful, almost psychedelic experience can fully purify and cleanse your body, mind, and spirit.

The Kundalini awakening is only the first step in the journey. This journey to connection and holistic wellness for yourself is one of the goals of Reiki as well. Since they have the same goal and a strong energetic component, both sources of energy work well together.

A Kundalini awakening can so profoundly change your life that it is recommended you pursue it with the guidance of a teacher or Master and that you are serious as a spiritual practitioner and healer.

There are some signs that indicate you have had a Kundalini awakening, so if you are wondering if you've experienced such an event, take a look at the signs below.

One

Everything falls apart, you have an emotional breakdown, and your old life isn't working.

This process of realization can feel or look similar to a midlife crisis. It can also be a point where you have a moment of clarity in which you need to change something, give up alcohol, leave your job, go back to school, whatever that sudden realization is, it will hit you hard!

Two

You'll experience symptoms that are physical, emotional, and energetic.

Some obvious symptoms can be shaking, intense stress, or near-death experiences. Other symptoms can include depression and anxiety. Essentially, at this point, the energy that is moving through the body and being released is too intense for the nervous system to handle. It gets completely overloaded.

Sometimes, the experience can be slow and steady. Other times, it can be fast and intense and hit you immediately. Rather than focusing on the symptoms, find ways to release blockages in the body to keep that energy moving and releasing what needs to be released.

Three

Courage, desire, and willingness to have new experiences.

Some people will experience an intense desire to change their diet, seek out a new job, or look for spiritual teachers or healers as a way to cope with or come to terms with what is happening internally.

When what you know stops working, your body and mind push for change and new experiences.

Four

You begin to receive support and answers from unexpected places. Miracles and synchronicities become obvious.

The point of desperation comes when we are open to trying new things and having new experiences. This is going to be when the mind and soul are open to receiving support from new places as well. This could come in the form of an unexpected teacher or a suggestion from a friend that you might have written off as silly prior to these experiences.

Your mind will begin to connect the dots between various events that seem miraculous but are really guiding you in an unexpected way.

Five

Increased sensitivity. Especially to external sources like people, places, media, and food.

With the changes that you begin to make in your life, body, and mind, your body will become more sensitive. You will be more in tune with yourself, thus allowing that same awareness and sensitivity to spread through the rest of your life and experiences.

Maybe you'll realize you need to leave a toxic relationship that didn't seem toxic before. Your body might urge you to eat cleaner foods by feeling sick any time you eat something processed. You might find it more difficult to watch violent TV shows, or feel more strongly about political situations.

Six

Intuition and truth that comes with the awareness of internal energies.

By becoming aware of what we need, we do turn into our own healers, just like with Reiki self-treatments. You'll become more aware and sensitive to everything around you, and everything within you.

You'll start to pay more attention to your own intuition. You'll care less about what other people think of you or say about you. This is the process in which you start to develop a relationship with your own soul.

It is important during this time to set aside time every day to work with your own energy. Meditation, yoga, and Reiki self-treatments are great ways to work with your own energy.

Seven
Increase in compassionate feelings, the desire to be helpful, and recognizing your own oneness.

Through your own experiences, you have gained knowledge and wisdom, and now you want to share that knowledge and wisdom with others. You'll naturally start to settle down into your new state of being. Once you begin to settle, sharing what you've learned and experienced with others is another natural reaction.

You'll connect with the earth, with your heart center, and with universal energy. Thus wanting to open up the people around you to the same connectedness and oneness.

Eight
You'll find your destiny, a sense of purpose.

Through this new connection and wisdom, you can begin to do what you came to this world to do. You will have found a strong sense of purpose for what you are meant to do. After you have healed your past, sorted through all the emotional baggage, conscious and unconscious, you can settle into your true self.

Are you meant to be a Reiki Master, a healer, a yoga teacher, an artist, a mother, whatever your true calling is, now is when you will feel it and understand it. The universe likes to support us when we finally begin to do what we are meant to do.

If you begin to experience a Kundalini awakening, whether you were expecting it or not, take some measures to ensure that it goes smoothly.

Steps to ease the awakening include:

- Purify the body (eat clean foods, avoid drugs and alcohol)
- Reduce Stress (Make time for the changes to happen, remove yourself from stressful situations and entanglements)
- Find Support (Find a teacher or community that can provide support from experience)
- Educate Yourself (Read about Kundalini and awakenings)
- Treat any Underlying Psychological Issues (Kundalini brings up anything that isn't

resolved. Getting help during the awakening with issues as they arise is recommended)

- Examine your own Spirituality (If you haven't already, it might be time to start meditating, taking a yoga class or other spiritual practices)
- Practice Grounding Rituals (Ground yourself daily to balance energy flow)

Reiki is an instrumental tool in calmly and gently promoting a Kundalini awakening. Kundalini Reiki is its own modality with its own Attunements, however, you do not need to be Attuned for Kundalini Reiki for Reiki to assist in a Kundalini awakening.

Since a Kundalini awakening is so powerful, it can cause turmoil and intense changes in a short period of time, especially if you aren't entirely ready for the awakening.

Performing daily self-treatments with Reiki is going to continue to smooth the Kundalini awakening as those Reiki treatments will help address stress, past issues, and unaddressed energy blockages. You might want to give yourself longer treatments, 60 minutes or more.

If you are attuned to Level II Reiki, including the Reiki symbols in your treatments are going to provide additional stability for the Kundalini awakening.

Doing Reiki meditation, especially the chakra clearing meditation, is going to promote a smoother flow of that Kundalini energy through your spine and chakras. Try to include the chakra and spine clearing meditation daily during a Kundalini awakening.

Including crystals that are associated with the Root chakra in Reiki meditations or treatments are also going to help by keeping the Root chakra stable and providing a grounded foundation to balance the Kundalini energy as it moves up through the spine.

If clients come to you who are experiencing a Kundalini awakening, providing them with Reiki treatments is also going to ease their transition. You will want to provide them with chakra work and grounding work during their Reiki treatments.

Reiki is a spiritual practice that reduces stress, helps ground the body, and clears the chakras, it can heal past traumas and unaddressed psychological issues and purify the body of toxins. Using Reiki during a Kundalini awakening meets many of the requirements on the list of steps to take for a smooth awakening. This makes it an ideal support tool during a Kundalini awakening.

Chapter Seven: Testimonials and Stories

Perhaps you're wondering if all of the information you have read can be backed up by real-life experiences. The following stories and testimonials are experiences that real people have had. They are documented instances from Reiki recipients, practitioners, and even casual observers.

This first story is an instance in which a pet owner witnessed his girlfriend performing Reiki on their pet ferret when she was sick.

"I've never been a believer in Reiki or energy work. I still don't really understand it. When our ferret, Angel, got sick, she was lethargic, excessively drooling, and her eyes were glazed over. It was late at night and we were considering rushing to the emergency vet. For over a half-hour we sat on the couch with Angel and watched her suffer.

I started to play video games to keep myself calm and that is when my girlfriend started doing Reiki on our ferret. I didn't know what she was doing at first, but then I saw her draw some symbols over Angel and assumed it was Reiki. In just minutes, Angel stopped drooling and started to stretch. After only five minutes, Angel was back to her wiggly, energetic self!

I can only describe what I saw as miraculous.

Over the next few months, there were more instances where Angel would become lethargic, start to drool and become weak, and have glazed eyes. Whether she was in that state for ten minutes or over an hour, just five minutes of Reiki from my girlfriend would completely return Angel to her normal energy levels!

It was truly incredible and gave us several more months with our beloved Angel."

-   Kristopher

Reiki is a powerful healing modality for both people and animals. A man who has no previous interest or belief in Reiki witnesses its healing power and then describes it as miraculous. Even without understanding how it works or what happened, he could visibly see the change it made in his pet when she was sick.

The next story we come to is from a Reiki Master who runs a private bodywork practice and sees clients for Massage, Reiki, and Shamanic work. It is the story of an experience she had with a specific client.

"Many of my massage clients know that I also offer Reiki sessions and Shamanic Healing sessions. One of my regular clients has been coming to see me for weekly 2-hour massages for over a year. He has asked me about Reiki on several occasions, so finally, when he had the time, he decided to get a Reiki session and try it out.

After the session, we discussed what he had felt or experienced. He said he didn't experience much, but he did see a lot of shades of purple during the session. As we wrapped up our day, I told him that some people will feel the effects of Reiki immediately while other people won't notice anything until later. I also said that Reiki isn't for everyone and some people try it out and decide that they don't want to continue with treatments for whatever reason.

He told me that he thinks that he is the kind of person who doesn't think he will get any benefit out of Reiki. I was disappointed, but I didn't push the matter.

When this client came to see me for his weekly massage a few days later, he was very excited to tell me about his follow up experience after our Reiki session. He told me that when he went home, he felt more energized than he had in a long time! He said that he was able to get so many projects around the house done that the felt like there wasn't enough time in the day to keep working. He never felt worn out or tired.

Then, later in his workweek, there were two days where changes were made to his workload and schedule that normally would have caused him anger and stress. He said that rather than getting mad, he was able to just go with the flow and keep a positive mindset.

My client attributed both of these experiences to the Reiki session. He still comes to see me for 2-hour massages once a week, but now, he will often get combo sessions of both Reiki and massage.

To this day, I haven't had a client who has received a Reiki session and then not felt any benefit or been interested in getting another one."

- Isabella

Since Reiki is subtle energy, sometimes, it can take time for the effects to be apparent. Educating your clients, as this Reiki Master did, is a good way to ensure that they know what to expect before and after a session.

This client didn't feel anything related to the Reiki session on the table but was aware enough to notice changes in his everyday life after the fact. Thus he could report back to his practitioner that he had experienced the benefit of Reiki and wanted to keep getting treatments.

The next story comes from a woman who had never heard of Reiki, but when her sister became a Reiki practitioner, she wanted to try it out and see what it was all about. She had gotten massages and spa treatments before, but she had never received energy work.

"I asked my sister to give me a Reiki session because I had never heard of it before but I figured I could try it out. I wanted to be supportive of what my sister was doing. I told her that I had been feeling very stressed about work and that I wanted to lose weight.

As soon as my sister started the session and put her hands on my head, I immediately felt like my entire brain was opening up. It was a very strange sensation. I just kind of let myself relax into the feeling because I was instantly relaxed by the work. All my stress just drained right away!

As my sister continued working, I realized that I had absolutely no awareness of my feet. Whatever normally connected my brain to the knowledge that my feet existed was just gone! It felt like they weren't there at all. It was strange, but not unsettling. Then when she got to my lower abdomen she drew a couple symbols on my body.

After the session, I told her how I had felt and she explained to me what to expect and how I might experience vivid dreams. She also cautioned me to drink plenty of water.

I returned home with my husband a few days later and resumed my normal life. I hadn't given much thought to my Reiki session until my husband pointed out that I hadn't been eating as big of portions at mealtimes. So I checked my weight and in only a week, I had lost around seven pounds! I hadn't even been consciously trying.

Now, I don't know if that was a subconscious placebo effect, but it worked. Whatever it was really worked. I hadn't even thought to keep track of my experiences until my husband made a comment. He hadn't even known I wanted to lose weight as one of the goals of my Reiki session. It wasn't like he was looking for weight-related results afterward.

I encouraged my sister to keep going with her Reiki practice because honestly, she made me a believer in the concept of energy work and I think she has a great gift to offer other people as well."

- Olivia

Another story in which someone who doesn't have previous experience with energy work, and who might be a little skeptical, but had a transformative experience on the table. This woman's experience during the session was much more profound, and then she continued to receive benefits after the fact. Even when she hadn't been keenly focused on her session, another outside observer was the first to notice a change.

The following story is another story about an animal who was receiving Reiki. The story comes from the pet's owner who was present at every treatment session.

"My baby boy was diagnosed with thyroid cancer. My husband and I decided that we wanted to go with a holistic approach to treating him. We didn't want him to go through painful treatments or be in and out of veterinary hospitals for months at a time. So, a friend of ours got us in touch with a local Reiki practitioner who worked on animals.

Not only did our Reiki practitioner come to meet us and our dog first for a free consultation, but every session, she came right to our house. The free consultation allowed us to determine if she would be a good match to work with our dog, and she was! Then having her come to our home meant our boy could be comfortable and relaxed during his sessions.

We started getting biweekly treatments for our dog. He was on a lot of other supplements and holistic medications for treatment. It was comforting to know that the Reiki energy wouldn't interfere with his other treatments.

Right away, we noticed differences in our dog. Whenever she started a Reiki session, he would come right up to her and want to be next to her. He would try to get in her lap or just roll over and want her to touch him all over. He was so happy when she started working. Then he would get up and go lie down under his favorite table and completely pass out.

Our other dog, a thirteen-year-old lab who has never been that keen on strangers or cuddling, would then go up to our Reiki practitioner and start licking her hands and sit right up against her.

It was so strange to see our lab being so affectionate and cuddly with someone she hardly knew! She must have sensed the energy.

Our Reiki practitioner began doing joint sessions on both our dogs. She would also use Reiki energy to clear our home and create a safe, relaxed space. My husband and I were present for all the sessions and we could really feel the difference in the atmosphere of our home. On the off weeks that we didn't have a session scheduled, we got in the habit of holding that same healing space for both our dogs at the same of day.

Over the months, we saw that our lovable baby boy would get so excited when our Reiki practitioner came over. He would run out to greet her and roll over and want her to touch him and pet him. It was great to see because we could tell that he was getting sicker. His energy levels weren't as high and his playfulness was waning, but seeing his reaction to her every time she came over was completely heartwarming.

We worked with a holistic vet as well who also told us that the tumor growth had slowed drastically since he had been receiving Reiki sessions.

My husband and I are so thankful that we found a Reiki practitioner who gave us several more good months with our baby."

- Holly

While Reiki isn't a cure-all, it can still be powerful in treating terminal illnesses, or at least, reducing the symptoms, as this woman witnessed in her dog. Reiki is a complementary treatment that can be used alongside other treatments, therapies, medications, and supplements without any interference. This applies to both working with people and animals. Reiki has been known to be especially effective when treating cancer patients to relieve pain and the side effects of treatments.

In many cases with cancer treatments, the patients are lacking something as simple as physical touch.

Having Reiki performed on them gives them a healing benefit and also provides them with physical contact. On a psychological level, that can be monumentally beneficial to patients being treated for invasive or terminal illnesses.

Our last story is from a woman who has traveled the world and had many different kinds of energy work and healing performed on her. She gets biweekly massages and biweekly Reiki sessions.

"I've experienced some incredible modalities over the years. When I found my Reiki practitioner though, everything for me changed. She brought my health and wellness to an entirely new level. I have received Reiki before and I've always been a little particular about who works on me, but when I found this practitioner, I knew right away that she was the perfect fit for me.

I have been struggling with a lot of health problems for years. Problems in my hips, low back, neck, and adrenal glands. When I started getting Reiki, the pain immediately began to release.

Unfortunately, the relief would only last for a few days, so I balanced Reiki and massage. But every time I went in for a Reiki session, I would learn something new.

I had also been dealing with major changes in my personal life. I wasn't quite sure where I wanted to go or how I was going to move forward. Not only was I looking for relief from physical pain, but I was also needing direction and guidance on a more personal level.

The biggest struggle I was having was in deciding whether or not I wanted to change or leave a job that I'd had for years. It was no longer fulfilling and I felt like it was sucking the life out of me.

The practitioner I found was not only a skilled healer but would talk to me about everything she found during a session and anything she saw or felt. We would discuss in length the things she saw as well as the things that

I would see. My mind would really travel when she worked on me.

It only took a couple of sessions with her for me to find the clarity I needed to change the course of my own life. The anxiety I had been feeling about leaving my job vanished and I knew it was the right course of action. I was finally able to move on with my own life and my own passions. I never would have had that without getting Reiki sessions.

After one session, my practitioner told me that she discovered a strong energy sensation in my C4 and C5 vertebrae. I had been experiencing worsening neck pain for a few weeks. With that information, I went to my doctor and they determined that I had begun developing arthritis in my C4 and C5 vertebrae. My whole neck had been hurting, but having my practitioner narrow down the source of the pain is what led me to seek out medical advice and now I have additional options for relieving my neck pains.

During my Reiki sessions, I began to notice that my breathing would change. Not only would I become more relaxed, but the pattern of my breathing would change. I mentioned this to my practitioner and she was able to keep a better eye on it. After a few more sessions, we talked about the changes in breathing.

Through our discussion and what I knew of my own family medical history, I thought it best to get tested for sleep apnea. It turned out I did have the preliminary development of sleep apnea. I was able to get on top of that development thankfully. Without Reiki, I wouldn't have been made aware of that odd change in my breathing and the sleep apnea could have gone along a lot longer without being addressed.

Additionally, as I kept going through my Reiki sessions, I was able to confront a lot of emotional baggage that I had been holding on to in regards to my own family. It was such a help to me physically and emotionally. I also made huge strides in my own medical treatments for a healthier lifestyle."

- *Deb*

Coming from a recipient that received long term, regular Reiki treatments really outlines how beneficial it can be on multiple levels of healing and improving lifestyle.

Conclusion

Thank you for reading through to the end of this book, *Reiki for Beginners*. Hopefully, you received the information that you wanted from reading this book. Your knowledge on the subject of Reiki should be expanding and giving you the foundation to continue your Reiki journey.

Now that you have finished reading this beginner's guide, it is time for you to decide where you want to take your Reiki journey. If you don't already have a Reiki Master to teach you, that'll be your first task on your new path. You have all the knowledge you need to decide where to take your journey next.

With the information provided in this book, you are ready to take your Reiki studies to the next level. Perhaps you are ready to study a specific area of interest, like Crystal Reiki, Reiki for Animals, or Kundalini Reiki.

Take some time to try out the exercises and meditations that have been provided in this book to better help you connect to universal energy and Reiki. As you progress on your journey, remember that these mediations and exercises are hugely beneficial to your studies and your understanding of Reiki.

Wherever your Reiki studies take you, thank you again for purchasing and reading this book. Your support is greatly appreciated. Please continue your journey with light and gratitude.

As a final note, if you did enjoy this book and felt that you gained important and new knowledge, please leave a review on Amazon. Your feedback is always appreciated!